BREAKING BAD EATING HABITS

3 CRUCIAL STEPS TO HELP YOU STOP DIETING,
INCREASE MINDFULNESS AND CHANGE YOUR LIFE -
AT ANY AGE

NICK SWETTENHAM

CONTENTS

STEP THREE. PRACTICAL
SOLUTIONS

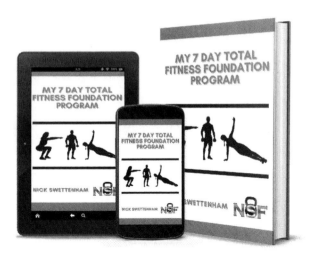

A Special Gift for my Readers

Included with the purchase of this book is My 7 Day Total Fitness Foundation Program to help you get started on your fitness journey. This program is a great way to start or adapt your training using all my 7 foundations. These foundations are:

1. Strength
2. Flexibility
3. Mobility
4. Stability
5. Agility
6. Endurance
7. Nutrition

Scan the QR code below and let us know the email address you would like it delivered to.

www.nickswettenhamfitness.com

INTRODUCTION

---

*"We cannot solve our problems with the same thinking
we used when we created them"*

— ALBERT EINSTEIN

Here we go again.

You're about to get started on the diet that will finally
propel you to your fat loss goals. At the same time, it
will balance out your nutritional deficiencies, cure your
gut problems and maximize your energy levels. You've
been here before, of course – but this time, it's different. You're determined and failure is not an option! It
will require a lot of pain, dedication and sacrifice, but

you're up to the task – there will be no more cheating, quitting or excuses.

But you will fail.

Just like you have failed every other time, you've followed the traditional diet-based method to weight loss. The raw truth is that it doesn't matter how determined, dedicated or devoted you are if the foundation is flawed. And the foundation upon which the western world bases its weight control and healthy nutrition guidance is seriously flawed. That's why we are in the midst of an obesity epidemic that is threatening to drown us all in a sea of fat.

The way we eat is not dictated by science, logic or nutritional expert guidance. We may think it is but we're fooling ourselves. The real drivers of what we put into our mouths are deeply ingrained habits that begin to form during our first year of life. By the time we move out of our parent's house and set up on our own, our way of eating, the times, quantities, food selections, amounts, and speed of eating are cemented into our routine. Even if we come to the realization that some of those habits are not good for our health, our efforts to change them will be sabotaged. That's because those lifetime nutritional habits are not just part of our conscious being – they are also deeply ingrained into our subconscious.

Your subconscious mind is like the 90 percent of the iceberg that sits below the water. Even though you may not be consciously aware of it, the subconscious is the controller of everything you do. It will give a measure of freedom to the conscious mind, but as soon as you try to overturn deeply ingrained subconscious habits, it will pull you back into line, doing whatever it can to disrupt your new way of doing things.

When it comes to food habits, the subconscious has a powerful ally. Eating, as you probably know all too well, has never been about simply supplying the machine which is your body with fuel in the form of calories. It is an intensely emotional experience. We eat in response to how we are feeling. When we're upset, we rush to the pantry for sugar-loaded comfort food. Then, when we're happy we celebrate with party food. Emotional urges work in tandem with our ingrained subconscious habits to ensure that whatever we do to get on top of our eating ends up a miserable failure.

So, does that mean that we should all throw in the towel, give up on the insane idea of getting healthy and resign ourselves to a forever fat future?

Well, you could do that - but there is a better way.

And that better way is what this book is all about.

It's the reason I have decided to add yet another book on nutrition to a saturated market. As a personal trainer, I work at the coalface of the nutritional nightmare every day. Most of the people I coach are confused, mystified and frustrated at all of the conflicting and nonsensical information they receive in answer to the seemingly simple question, "What should I eat?"

Helping you achieve optimal health through sensible nutrition matters deeply to me because I, like you, have found achieving the right nutritional lifestyle challenging. It is a journey we all go through in life and the destination has taken time and effort to reach.

Over my years of working with hundreds of clients, I have discovered that there are 3 fundamental steps to achieving nutritional success. Whether your goal is to lose body fat, build lean muscle, get rid of gut problems, achieve optimal energy and health, or a combination of all of these. Here they are . . .

Step 1 – Identifying habits throughout our lives and understanding why these have manifested.
Step 2 – Change our mindset and learn how to break those habits through self-reflection, honesty and mindful eating techniques.
Step 3 – Implement practical knowledge solu-

tions to provide you with a detailed basic education in nutrition., along with practical tips and meal ideas.

The book you are about to read is set out in harmony with those 3 steps.

Chapters 1-4 explore the habits that have shaped the way we eat. We will come to understand how our upbringing and parental habits can shape not only our eating habits from a young age but also from pre-birth. Societal issues that help shape bad habits and that we use as excuses not to change will also be uncovered. We will also explore how aging and stress affect the way we eat. In this section, you will also discover why the diets that you may have been relying on in the past will never work - in fact, they will actually make you fatter!

Chapters 5 and 6 are where we begin to implement practical solutions so that you can break out of the eating habit trap. You will discover how to change your mindset, so you are able to create new rules that are guilt-free and easier to maintain a healthy lifestyle.

Our final section, Chapters 7-9, presents a treasure trove of practical solutions. You will learn of the importance of food as energy, as well as the role of hydration and recovery in combating issues like stress that can lead to bad habits. I will also present a no-

nonsense, easy to understand grounding in nutrition, macro and micronutrients so you can feel confident going forward. We conclude with a bunch of ideas, tips and recipes to help you form better eating habits.

By the time you reach the end of this book, you will finally have the solution to the problem that has been sabotaging your efforts to get on top of nutrition. You will have gained the knowledge to overcome bad eating habits, ditched the dieting dilemma, optimized the way you eat with newer, better habits, and changed your life forever.

STEP ONE. IDENTIFYING HABITS

1

PRE-BIRTH NUTRITION, PARENTAL AND SOCIETAL INFLUENCE

"It isn't where you came from. It's where you're going that counts"

— ELLA FITZGERALD

NUTRITION DURING PREGNANCY

We have known for a long time that the foods we give our children and the messages we expose them to have an impact on their adult nutritional habits. Recent research, however, has revealed that parental influence on the way we eat goes back further than we ever expected. In fact, even before we take our first breath, the choices that our mother makes about what she puts in her mouth have an effect on us.

A 2008 study that was published in the journal *Science News* showed that poor nutritional choices made by pregnant women could put their baby at risk of developing long-term, irreversible health issues. These include obesity, increased HDL cholesterol concentrations and increased blood sugar levels. The study showed that the effects were more pronounced on females than on males.

Not only does the baby's experience in the womb affect its future health, but it is a determining factor in all areas of life, including future eating habits. A long-term research program known as the Developmental Origins of Health and Disease showed that the first 1,000 days of an individual's existence, counted from the moment of conception, were hugely impactful on the life of that child. Poor nutritional choices on the part of the mother can negatively impact the developing baby's development of organs and hormonal and metabolic responses.

The first month after conception is considered to be a crucial window during which it is most important that the mother eats a healthy, balanced diet. Of course, many women are not even aware that they're pregnant at this stage. This is one reason why prospective parents would do well to plan for pregnancy, with the female partner eating as if she were pregnant as a normal state of being. Their partner can also help by adopting these habits as support.

Each of the organs of the human body has a critical period of development. If there is a lack of nutrients due to poor food choices by the mother, the organ will be compromised. For example, if the fetus is poorly nourished when the kidneys develop, fewer nephrons will be produced. Their job is to filter blood. For the rest of that child's life, he or she will struggle to perform that vital function adequately.

Healthy eating during pregnancy includes eliminating processed foods and focusing on nutrient-dense foods. Here are nine nutrients to focus on during pregnancy:

- Folate
- Vitamin C
- Zinc
- Iron
- Fatty Acids
- Calcium
- Vitamin B12

- Vitamin D
- Choline

Prenatal nutrition even has an effect on our genetic make-up. Our basic genetic structure does not change, but environmental factors can make changes to the way our genes express themselves. An example of this was seen in the Netherlands during the Second World War, when famine led to a large number of malnourished pregnant women. This resulted in an adjustment in the epigenetic process known as DNA methylation in the offspring. These genetic expression adaptations predisposed the babies to later metabolic problems, elevated blood sugar levels, increased body mass index and higher LDL cholesterol levels.

In the last couple of decades, obstetricians have become increasingly alarmed at a new trend - obese babies. To have a baby come out of the womb weighing as much as 12 pounds is no longer a rarity. Hundreds of babies are born every year in the UK who are classified as being obese; that means that they weigh more than 9 lbs, 15 oz at birth.

As a result of the increasing fatness of babies, more and more women are being forced to have caesarean sections because the baby is too large to come out of the womb.

While it is true that some of these obese babies have piled on the pounds because their mothers suffer from a medical disorder, the vast majority are due to mothers eating too much. According to Tam Fry of the UK National Obesity Forum, "It is believed that 82 percent of children who are obese will continue to be overweight. As they had the same kind of nutrition as their parents, there is a continual spiral upwards."

CHILDHOOD INFLUENCES

Every baby starts out drinking mother's milk. But after that, it's all where you happen to have been born. If your first breath took place on the plains of Tanzania, post-milk nutritional experience would kick off with bone marrow from wild game. If you were born in the Far Eastern Republic of Laos, that first food would be gelatinous rice that has been pre-chewed by your mother and transferred from her mouth to yours. If you happen to be a western baby, your first bite of solid food is likely to be powdered cereal from a packet or puree from a jar. Those foods that are introduced early are the ones that will likely ingrain themselves as part of our eating habits.

None of us are born with an inbuilt knowledge of how and what to eat. These things have to be taught by our parents. From them, we learn what foods satisfy our hunger and provide us with the energy we need to function. We also learn when to stop eating. In former times, parents exposed their babies to a wide variety of food choices. However, over the past hundred years, those food choices have become far more homogenous.

During the first couple of years of life, our parents are the main determinants of our food choices. But from then onward, that decision making has increasingly been overtaken by food conglomerates. From as early as 2 years of age, children are continually exposed to food companies that are pushing foods that are high in sugar, saturated fats and salt. The youngster then puts pressure on their parents to feed them those foods. The addictive nature of high carb foods soon kicks in and the kid is soon unable to go through the day without their 'fix'.

Meanwhile, the food companies are coming up with ever more inventive ways to cash in children's longing for foods that nurture unhealthy eating habits.

The realization that our adult eating practices are shaped by the habits we learn as children should give us pause to rethink some of the things we have been doing with our kids. Think about eating vegetables. When we feel the need to hide carrots or brussels sprouts in other, more tempting foods, we are sending a strong message to our kids. We are telling them that vegetables are bad. Is that really what you want your kids to think? I don't think so.

Children are like sponges. They are always watching, analyzing and making conclusions. They do it about food perhaps more frequently than anything else. While a lot of what the child absorbs is conscious - like what to eat, when to eat it and when to stop - a surprising amount is subconscious. This includes the idea that, while vegetables are necessary, they are like an unpleasant medicine that has to be tolerated and that the good foods (in the sense of delighting the taste buds) are what we reward ourselves with when we want to celebrate and what we comfort ourselves with when we feel depressed.

Our basic food preferences, such as sweet or salty flavors are genetically predetermined. However, these genetic predispositions are modified by experience during childhood. The influence of parents in this process is huge. Research has shown that certain parental practices, such as exerting too much control over what and how much the child eats can contribute to the child being overweight. In their attempts to prevent children from having access to junk foods and pressuring them to eat healthy foods, many parents cause a negative rebellious reaction that sees the child eating more than other children of those 'forbidden fruit' foods as they develop a little more freedom in their pre-teens and teens. This often led to the child becoming overweight. Researchers conclude that it is much better to teach children by good parental example rather than imposing restrictions on them.

In the family environment, there is a wide interplay of factors that affect a child's perceptions around food. These include:

- The weight of the parents
- The parent's personal food choices
- Portion sizes
- Amount and types of food available at home
- Frequency of eating out
- Time of consumption
- Temperature and smell of foods
- Eating at the dinner table vs in front of the TV
- Physical activity
- The use of food as a reward
- The use of food as a comfort

Often, for the first year or two of a child's life, the parents are very mindful of what they feed their young-ster. But then, as mum goes back to work, life gets busier and, often other kids come along, pre-child eating habits are reverted to. Setting a good example to the young one takes a back seat to the practicalities of life.

Here are 9 bad eating habits that kids pick up from their parents:

1. Salting food before tasting it - excessive salt consumption is a big problem, leading to high blood pressure and water retention.
2. Eating too fast - eating on the run is one of the root causes of overeating. That's because we don't give our body time to realize that it is full before the next mouthful enters the stomach. As a result, we are teaching our kids not to listen to their hunger cues! Eating on the run also denies the ability to savor and enjoy the abundant flavors in our foods, relegating eating to a purely mechanical process.
3. Skipping breakfast - mornings can get pretty hectic, making it difficult to find time to prepare breakfast. If we skip it, we are modeling that same behavior in our kids. Then, when they turn up at school without having topped up their fuel supply, they will lack focus in the classroom. By 11 am, they'll be desperate for sugary carbs, which they'll usually find at the school vending machine.
4. Overnight snacking - midnight snacking is a

surefire route to fat gain. Don't model it, even if you think the kids are sleeping. Instead, stop eating at least an hour before bedtime.

5. Avoiding vegetables - there's more to vegetables than mashed potatoes and a token bit of lettuce salad. If you tend to avoid vegetables, your kids will too. Parents who experiment with the wide variety of vegetables on offer are more likely to have kids who enjoy things like beets, butternut squash and zucchini.

6. Using food as a reward - having a sweet treat every now and then is fine, but when we reward ourselves, or our kids, with carb-loaded foods, we are sending them a powerful message; sugary foods are the jackpot! That message will very quickly become embedded into their subconscious.

7. Large portions - many kids who become overweight don't do so as a result of eating 'bad'; the problem is that they are eating too much food. The size of dinner plates has increased 30% since the 1950s. With most peoples' tendency being to fill the plate, it's hardly surprising that we are eating a whole lot more calories nowadays. So, rather than loading a large dinner plate and then telling your child that they have to eat everything

that's on it, go out and buy a set of smaller plates and allow the child's natural hunger cues to dictate when they stop eating.

8. Not drinking enough water - if your child only sees you drinking coffee, soda, wine or beer, they are not going to be very inclined to drink water, no matter how much you harp on about it. Modeling high water consumption is one of the best nutrition habits you can instill in your kids.

9. Fast food reliance - When life gets hectic, it's easy to forego the kitchen and either order KFC delivered or pack everyone in the car and head down to your local burger joint. But, think about what you are teaching your kids. Fast food is the 'go-to' solution whenever you get busy. Imagine how much better your child will be prepared for adult life if he saw you meal prepping fresh food rather than simply pulling out ready to go meals from the freezer.

MEDIA INFLUENCE

I don't have to tell you that the media pushes unhealthy food on kids - they've been doing it for more than fifty years. Of course, food companies have to get their message out there, but that doesn't account for the fact that 97% of all food advertising is for what nutritionists consider to be unhealthy food. Food companies spend more than $2 billion every year directly pushing their message to children. That is $1.94 billion being spent annually convincing your kids to put stuff into their bodies that is bad for them!

Governments around the world have been very slow to regulate the marketing of unhealthy food to children. In 2006, the UK government took the lead by imposing statutory restrictions preventing advertising for foods high in fats, sugars and salts around programs that were created for children under the age of 16. As a result of this measure, by 2009, according to a UK Department of Health report, the annual expenditure for child-themed food and drink products fell by 41%.

Measures like this are positive. The problem, however, is that fewer and fewer kids are watching TV. They are all online. And the food companies have complete free reign to push their high sugar, high fat and high sodium foods on social media platforms. As a result, we see more kids spending more hours sitting on their butts staring at a screen that is constantly enticing them with bad food. And then we wonder why we are in the midst of a childhood obesity epidemic!

How does all of this screen time exposure to food affect us? A study out of the University of Pittsburgh School of Medicine showed that study participants who spent the most time on social media were 2.6 times more likely to report problems with body image and eating than those who spent minimal time in front of the computer.

Another powerful influence on eating habits, especially as children enter their pre-teen years, is peer pressure. Research shows that more than three-quarters of pre-teens will make food choices when eating out that are in line with the preferences of their friends. Contrast this with the 40+ age group, in which just 2.7 percent of people will make fast food choices as a result of perceived peer pressure.

The food marketers take advantage of peer influence by constructing marketing campaigns to make kids feel they are missing out or that they're not part of the 'in' crowd if they don't buy their food product.

WHAT ABOUT EATING DISORDERS?

Eating disorders such as anorexia and bulimia nervosa are the result of complex and poorly understood causes. Sexual and mental abuse, parental conflict, pressure from sports coaches and the influence of society's ideals of body shape have all been implicated.

The eating disorder sufferer falls into a cycle of depression and low self-esteem, which they express through an obsession with their weight. Once they start to link body image and eating with mood and self-esteem, a cycle of extreme dieting and or/ bingeing and subsequent self-loathing can result.

They may see weight loss as the solution to their problems and feel that exerting strict control over their diet will help them control their emotional difficulties. All eating disorders are potentially dangerous. Sufferers are unlikely to help themselves and often deny having a problem. Most treatments emphasize both nutritional and psychological counseling.

SUMMARY

By the time we have moved out of our parent's home and are out on our own, we have all developed the habits that are going to drive our nutritional future. Those habits are an amalgam of all the things we have discussed in this chapter. For many of us, the combination of prenatal nutrition, cultural differences, food company advertising, parental example, social media influences, peer pressure, and societal pressures to look a certain way have resulted in bad nutritional habits that have put us in a place where we do not want to be.

In our next chapter, we explore the effect that poor nutritional choices have on the aging process. After revealing how bad food choices can speed up the aging process, we then drill down on the key anti-aging foods you need to focus on helping fight the effects of aging.

2

HOW BAD NUTRITION AFFECTS THE AGING PROCESS

"My belief is that it's a privilege to get older. Not everybody gets to be older"

— CAMERON DIAZ

Many people dread the aging process. After the age of 40, they view each coming birthday as one more marker that their body is declining, the vitality ebbing away and the march toward the grave quickening.

Then there are others who have a completely different view.

As they progress into their 40s, 50s and beyond, they view themselves as getting better, stronger and more energetic with each passing day. They accept, of course, that they are not immune to certain age-related physical changes, but they are not ruled by them. In fact, they accept them as a challenge and look for ways to minimize their effect so that they can retain their youthful vigor and enjoy life to the full.

Often the difference between the two comes down to nutrition.

In this chapter, we break down what happens to the body as we age and how our nutrition choices can either exacerbate or ameliorate that process.

HOW THE BODY CHANGES AS WE AGE

Fat Accumulation

The older you get, the harder it is to lose weight. From the age of 30, your metabolism steadily declines. That means that your body burns fewer calories. So, even if your activity level in your 40s is the same as it was in your 20s, you will still have a much harder time losing weight. That's one reason why it's so important to make smart food choices as we get older.

Allergies

As we age, we may find ourselves becoming allergic to things that did not affect us previously. Dairy is one of the most common allergies to emerge in later life. Many people in their 40s develop lactose intolerance. Your body creates lactase, an enzyme that digests lactose. But, as you age, your body produces less lactase, which makes it difficult to break down the lactose in dairy foods. This can result in bloating, headaches, diarrhea, gas and skin breakouts.

Plaque Build-Up

As we age, a build-up of cholesterol tends to line the arteries, making it increasingly difficult for blood to flow correctly. This could result in a blood clot or even a heart attack.

Reducing Perspiration

The older you get, the less you sweat. Women experience this more than men as a result of menopausal hormone changes. Sweat glands shrink and become less sensitive.

Reduced Muscle Mass

All people lose muscle mass as they get older. The muscles also lose their elasticity. Age-related muscle loss is called sarcopenia. From the age of 30 onward, men will lose between 3-5 percent of their muscle mass every decade. Reduced muscle mass makes a person weaker and reduces their functional mobility.

Brain Shrinkage

As we age, certain parts of the brain shrink. The most affected parts of the brain are those associated with learning and complex mental activities. Communication between neurons in parts of the brain is also negatively affected by aging. In addition, reduced neural blood flow and inflammation impair cognitive function.

As a result of age-related brain factors, older people may find it more challenging to recall names or other familiar information, having difficulty multitasking and a reduced attention span.

Reduced Tooth Sensitivity

As you age, the nerves in your teeth shrink. As a result, not only do your teeth become less sensitive, but you may be unaware if you have dental problems such as a cavity. That's why it's important to maintain a schedule of regular dental check-ups as you age.

Skin Changes

As you age, your skin becomes thinner, loses fat and produces more oil. This results in drier and less elastic skin. The number of nerve endings in the skin is also reduced, which results in reduced skin sensitivity. Older people also have fewer skin melanocytes, which makes them more susceptible to the effects of ultraviolet radiation.

Hair Quantity and Quality

As we age, we lose hair pigment cells, known as melanin. That's why our hair begins to turn grey. It also becomes thinner on the scalp, more frequently with men than women. As we age, our hair follicles produce thinner, smaller hairs. In time, they may produce none at all.

Loss of Height

We begin losing height in our 30s. Over the course of a lifetime, men can shrink about an inch, while women may lose double that. Height loss is the result of changes in bones, muscles and joints.

Urinary Function

The aging process is not kind to the bladder. It becomes weaker with the result that, as we age, we need to visit the bathroom more often. Uncontrollable bladder issues are also common as we age.

Facial Changes

In our 20s, our facial skin is rich in collagen and firm. From our 30s onward, the effects of sun exposure become evident. These include sunspots, wrinkles and dark patches on the forehead, cheeks and chin. In our 40's, facial skin is much drier, with prominent lines and wrinkles becoming etched in place. Subcutaneous facial skin reduces, often unevenly.

Heart Health

As we age, the heart begins to slow down in its activity. At the same time, arteries become stiffer. This combination of factors puts increasing pressure on the heart. This may cause the heart muscle to become enlarged. This is a contributing factor to heart disease.

Reduced Taste

By the age of 60, you will lose half of your taste buds. That's a big reason that older people seem to enjoy sweet treats more and tend to add a lot of salt to their food.

Hormonal Changes

Menopausal hormonal changes affect both men and women. This can make older people more susceptible to such conditions as diabetes, lupus and arthritis.

Menopause in men is called andropause and is characterized by a drop in testosterone production.

Aching Bones

The older you get, the more likely you are to suffer from aching bones. This is the result of general wear and tear on the machine that is your body. Bone density decreases as we age. This makes bones more brittle, which can lead to bone fractures. Osteoarthritis is an age-related bone condition.

Digestive Disorder

Around 40 percent of seniors suffer from an age-related digestive disorder. One of the most common is constipation. This is characterized by painful or infrequent bowel movements and hard, dry stools. Also common are slower muscle contractions in the digestive system, which causes food to move more slowly through the colon.

Older adults often take medication, which may cause digestive issues. After the age of 50, there is also an increased risk of developing polyps, which are small growths in the colon. Polyps may become cancerous.

Research reveals that 20 percent of seniors have a condition known as atrophic gastritis, which results in low levels of stomach acid. This makes it more difficult to absorb nutrients, especially Vitamin B12 and the minerals iron, magnesium and calcium.

CHANGING NUTRITIONAL NEEDS

As we age, our nutrition requirements evolve. In order to offset many of the natural consequences of aging that we have just examined, it becomes increasingly important to eat a more healthy diet. Here is a summary of the significant aging changes specifically related to nutrition:

- Low stomach acid makes it much harder to absorb nutrients
- Slower metabolism results in a reduced caloric need
- Taste sensation is compromised
- There is a reduced sensitivity to our sensations of hunger and thirst
- Digestive system disorders including constipation, urinary problems and bloating

These changes present a sort of Catch 22 situation for older people; they need to take in **more** nutrients to offset reduced absorption while at the same time consuming **fewer** calories. In order to achieve these apparently contradictory ambitions, it is vital to focus on nutrient-dense foods.

Age-related metabolic rate decline is the result of a combination of factors. One of them is the gradual loss of muscle mass that takes place as we get older. Muscles are 5 times more dense than fat. As a result, it requires a lot more energy to sustain. As you lose muscle, your metabolism will be reduced. Reduced activity levels also result in a slower metabolism.

Even if a person in their 50s or 60s were to have the exact same level of activity and the same amount of muscle as a person in their 20s, they would still have a lower metabolism. This was shown in a 2001 study conducted by the University of Colorado. However, this change will not be nearly as significant as when the older person does little exercise and does not control their diet. In the study, the older men burned 71.8 calories per hour compared with 73.8 for the younger men.

What this shows is that the two key lifestyle factors of exercise and controlled nutrition are the most important controllers of metabolism as we age.

Reducing caloric intake is especially important in aging women. That's because the hormonal changes that occur during menopause lead to a decline in estrogen levels that can result in belly fat storage.

In order to meet their nutrient needs while eating fewer calories, older people should focus on eating the following whole foods:

- Vegetables
- Fruits
- Lean Meats
- Fish

The most important nutrients that are needed as we age are Vitamin B12, Vitamin D, Calcium and Protein.

Taking in more protein will help to offset the natural decline in muscle mass that occurs with aging. A 2008 study followed the dietary habits of more than 2000 older people over 3 years. It was found that those who ate the most protein experienced an average 40 percent lower rate of muscle decline than those who ate less protein. Those who combined increased protein intake with a regular program of resistance exercise experienced an even more significant reduction in natural muscle mass loss.

Constipation is a common problem amongst the elderly population. In people over the age of 65, it is three times more common in women than in men. One contributing factor is the medications that older people are taking that have constipation as one of their side effects. In order to help alleviate this problem, older people should concentrate on increasing their fiber consumption. Fiber is digested by the body, passing through and helping you pass softer and larger stools.

There are two types of fiber:

- Soluble
- Insoluble

Soluble fiber is found in such foods as nuts, seeds, beans, lentils and some fruits and vegetables. Insoluble fiber comes from whole grains, vegetables and wheat bran.

The majority of foods that are high in fiber contain a blend of soluble and insoluble fiber. Insoluble fiber will provide bulk to your stools. It also flushes the waste through the bowels to form them into stools. Soluble fiber absorbs water to create a gel-like substance. That becomes part of the stool. This will promote greater passage of the stool through the bowels.

As we age, our bones naturally become weaker and more brittle. Increasing our intake of Calcium and Vitamin D is the key to offsetting these changes. Calcium will help to increase the bone mass, while Vitamin D will increase the body's enhancement of Calcium. That's important because older people have a reduced ability to absorb Calcium. Researchers believe that this is due more to reduced Vitamin D intake than any natural decline. Also, as the body ages, it does not produce as much Vitamin D.

In order to get more Calcium and Vitamin D, older people should include a rich supply of the following in their diet:

- Dairy products
- Green leafy vegetables
- Salmon
- Herring

Older people also need more Vitamin B12, also known as cobalamin. B12 is required for the manufacture of red blood cells and for cognitive functioning. Studies have shown that between 10-30 percent of people over the age of 50 have a reduced ability to absorb Vitamin B12. This vitamin is attached to proteins in food. Before the body can use it, it must first be detached from its proteins. However, reduced levels of stomach acid make this a problem for older people. That is why taking a Vitamin B12 supplement is a good idea for seniors. Eating foods that have been fortified with B12 is also beneficial, as the B12 contained in them is not bound to protein.

Good sources of Vitamin B12 are eggs, fish, meat and dairy products.

As we age, our sensitivity to the thirst sensation is reduced. Couple this with the fact that kidney function can also be compromised with age, and it's no surprise that many older people do not drink enough water. This reduces cell fluid levels. A direct effect of this for older people is that it is much harder to absorb the active ingredients in medications.

Getting into the habit of drinking one or two glasses of water before eating a meal rather than relying on the thirst sensation will help older people stay well hydrated.

Older people often experience a reduced desire to eat. Age-related decreased appetite can result in nutrient deficiencies and exacerbated muscle tissue loss. Research shows that seniors have higher levels of leptin, the hunger-suppressing hormone and lower levels of ghrelin, the hunger initiating hormone.

The reasons for reduced appetite as we age may include less sensitivity of taste and smell, medications that decrease the appetite and the loss of teeth.

People who have difficulty eating large meals should eat several smaller meals spaced throughout the day.

Eating nutrient-dense foods such as eggs, avocado, nuts and yogurt is also important.

9 FOODS THAT OLDER PEOPLE NEED TO REDUCE

As we age, it becomes even more important to avoid the foods we know we should steer clear of at any age. Here are the top 9 foods to cut back on.

Ice Cream, Candy & Cake

Sugar ages the body faster than any of the natural age declines we've discussed previously. Regularly eating it in the form of ice cream, candy and cake result in those sugars binding with protein. This has a negative impact on skin collagen, with the result that your skin loses its elasticity and youthfulness. Sugar also results in tooth discoloration and tooth decay.

Sugar, of course, is also the main culprit when it comes to unhealthy weight gain. Using natural sugar substitutes such as stevia and experimenting with natural fruit alternatives to sweet desserts will help you control your sweet urges.

Alcohol

Monitoring your alcohol intake is important at any age, but as we age, it becomes more critical. A healthy liver helps to eliminate toxins from the skin and other parts of the body. Excessive alcohol consumption, however, has a detrimental effect on the liver. Toxins that would otherwise be flushed from the body by the liver accumulate under the skin. This can lead to a prematurely aged look to the skin, swollen eyes, wrinkles and acne.

Alcohol also dehydrates the skin. This reduces the elasticity of the skin,as well as leading to patchiness, uneven pigmentation and dryness. It also destroys tooth enamel, which results in unattractive staining.

You don't have to become a teetotaler when you hit middle age, but you should cut down your intake. Moderation, as with most things, is the key to an enjoyable, healthy and long life.

Fried Foods & Sushi

Fried foods and sushi are very high in salt content, which causes water retention. This makes the skin appear puffy and bloated. Seniors should cut down on pre-cooked and preserved foods which are salt-heavy.

A diet that is high in salty foods increases the risk of high blood pressure and heart disease. It can also lead to excess Calcium in the urine, which increases the likelihood of developing kidney stones. Too much salt in the blood can also reduce blood flow to the heart and the brain. This increases the risk factor for heart attack and stroke. Researchers at the University of Maryland School of Medicine have estimated that a 50 percent reduction in salt content in restaurants and processed foods would save an estimated 150,000 lives per year.

Studies have also found that a diet rich in salty foods such as salty fish also increases the risk of gastric cancer.

Processed Meats

Processed meats such as sausages, corned beef, salami and ham contain lots of salts, preservatives and sulfites. These chemicals are known to trigger skin inflammation and accelerate the aging process. Processed meat is also one of the leading causes of heart disease, high blood pressure and respiratory complications.

The high amount of sodium in processed meats also contributes to puffiness and dehydration in the skin.

Char-Grilled Meats

Charred meat contains pro-inflammatory hydrocarbons, which cause damage to the collagen in the skin. That's why it is important to remove char from your grill after using the barbecue. When cooking meat, be careful not to over-grill it, as doing so could lead to the formation of skin-damaging free radicals.

You do not have to give up on red and white meats, as they provide an excellent source of protein. Just be sure to choose the leanest cuts possible and not overcook them. Pair them with green leafy vegetables that are rich in antioxidants.

Foods that Contain Trans Fats

Trans fats are a form of saturated fat. A trans fat is created when a vegetable oil undergoes the process of hydrogenation. This is done to extend the shelf life of the food by causing the food to harden at room temperature. Commercially fried foods, cookies, crackers and margarines all contain trans fats. Trans fats can make even unsaturated fats act like saturated fats. You need to avoid them at all costs.

Trans fats do not fold upon themselves in the way that other fats do. Unfortunately, this leads to an increased risk of coronary heart disease, cancer and many other chronic conditions. What's more, trans fats increase bad LDL cholesterol levels and lower good HDL cholesterol levels.

A high intake of trans fats has also been linked to an increased risk of Alzheimer's disease, lymphoma, liver cholesterol synthesis, and suppressing the excretion of bile acids.

Here are five foods that are high in trans fatty acids:

- French fries
- Margarine
- Fried chicken
- Onion rings
- Donuts

Spicy Foods

Spices can cause havoc with your pH levels. The skin's pH levels are particularly sensitive to spices. This will cause skin irritation and may cause acne outbreaks. Spicy foods will intensify skin blotches. People with rashes will usually experience outbreaks after eating spicy food, especially during menopause. During this period, the blood vessels become more sensitive and reactive. This increases the likelihood of damage to the blood vessels when you eat spicy foods.

Caffeine

Caffeine is a diuretic that depletes the body of fluid and moisture. This can cause dehydration of the skin, making it look aged and dull. If you have developed a sizable coffee drinking habit over your lifetime, try to switch to decaffeinated versions. Another strategy to reduce your caffeine consumption is to set the target of matching every cup of coffee with a glass of water. This will have the dual purpose of keeping your body hydrated and filling you up on healthy liquids.

Canned Soup

Canned soup is high in sodium, preservatives and added artificial flavors. All of these are bad for your body. As we've already discovered, excess sodium will dehydrate your body and cause water retention. This will result in puffy skin and more visible fine lines.

So long as you avoid the ready-made, canned variety, soups can actually prove an excellent, nutrient dense meal for anyone and particularly seniors who struggle to eat solid foods. A blender or food sieve is all that you need to turn everyday ingredients into a filling, healthy dish. Homemade soups have a distinct advantage over canned versions as they allow you to control the levels of salt and sugar, and to preserve nutrients that are lost in processing. Try pumpkin soup made with pumpkin, onion, nutmeg, a stock cube and some water. You could also substitute vegetables such as broccoli and carrots for the pumpkin.

9 FOODS THAT OLDER PEOPLE NEED TO INCREASE

Water

Keeping ourselves well hydrated is important at any age, but especially so over the age of 40. Your body is around 60% water, with the blood containing 90%. You should aim to consume about 2 L of water every day. The challenge as we get older is that our sensation for thirst decreases. That makes it all the more important to consciously think about meeting your daily requirements. Keeping up your H_2O intake will regulate your body temperature, help you think clearly, flush toxins from your body and help your muscles to contract strongly.

Broccoli

Broccoli is a super vegetable with both anti-inflammatory and anti-aging properties. As well as being packed with phytochemicals and high in protein, it is also full of antioxidants to combat free radical damage. In addition, broccoli is an excellent source of fiber. Maintaining a healthy fiber intake will not only keep you regular but help to control your appetite. Broccoli is a rich source of Vitamin C. Among its other benefits, vitamin C promotes the production of collagen to keep the skin looking vibrant. Broccoli is even good for your brain as it contains folate, Calcium and lutein, which have been linked to enhanced memory.

For maximum benefit, eat your broccoli raw. If you prefer to eat it cooked, steaming will best preserve its nutrients.

Blueberries

Blueberries have the highest antioxidant counts of all fruits and vegetables. In fact, they contain a special type of antioxidant called anthocyanins. These are responsible for the blue color of this berry and contain powerful anti-aging properties. They are great for improving heart health, reducing cholesterol, fighting obesity, and slowing down age-related brain functioning degeneration. They even help to prevent colds and flu.

Nuts

Snacking on nuts and adding them to your salads, oatmeal and smoothies is a great way to increase your healthy nutrient intake. Two of the best sources are almonds and walnuts. Almonds provide an excellent source of vitamin E, which allows your body to repair damaged skin tissue, keeps your skin hydrated and protects it from sun damage. Be sure to eat almonds with their skins, as that is what contains the vast majority of the antioxidants in this nut. Almonds have also been shown to help to reduce cognitive decline in seniors.

Walnuts are a great source of Omega 3 fatty acids, which have a powerful anti-inflammatory effect. They have also been shown to help reduce the risk of heart disease.

Watercress

In addition to providing an excellent source of hydration, watercress is extremely nutrient-dense. It is especially high in vitamins A, C, K, B1 and B12. It's packed with antioxidants to fight off oxidative stress. In addition, watercress boosts immunity, improves digestion and supports thyroid function.

Bell Peppers

Red and orange bell peppers are especially high in antioxidants. Red bell peppers have the highest vitamin C content, which helps to build collagen to keep your skin looking healthy. The bright colors of bell peppers are due to what are known as carotenoids. These contain powerful anti-inflammatory properties.

Bell peppers make a satisfying snack on their own, especially if dipped in hummus.

Spinach

Spinach is another vegetable that will improve your hydration while delivering a powerful antioxidant boost to your body. Just like red bell peppers, spinach is high in vitamin C. It's also an excellent source of vitamin A, which is great for hair health, and vitamin K, which helps fight off inflammation.

Avocado

Avocados are a genuine superfood. They contain healthy fatty acids that ward off inflammation in the body and promote healthy skin. They are also rich in carotenoids and vitamins A and E. These two vitamins will help to keep the skin looking youthful and nourished. The high levels of antioxidants and avocados make them among the best foods you can eat to counter the oxidative stress caused by free radicals.

Chickpeas

Chickpeas are an excellent source of protein. As we've discovered already, as we age, we need fewer calories but just as much, if not more, protein. Getting it through sources such as chickpeas is a smart way to go. They are very nutrient-dense and contain a high protein count for their calorie cost. As well as being a very good source of protein, chickpeas are also high in fiber, iron and copper.

Cutting back on red meat as your go to source for protein and increasing your intake of plant-based sources such as chickpeas, beans and legumes is a smart move for seniors.

AVOIDING WEIGHT GAIN AS YOU AGE

Many people gain weight as they age. However, research makes it clear that age-related weight gain is by no means inevitable. While the body's metabolic rate does slow down after the mid to late 30s, the main reason why people gain weight seems to be because they are not physically active and are eating too much food, regardless of how healthy that food happens to be.

For women, menopause also leads to changes in fat distribution. This is due to a drop in estrogen levels. At this time of life, fat begins to collect around the waist and on the stomach. By understanding that the body now needs fewer calories, you can make changes at the crucial time and prevent, or at least reduce, weight gain. Preventing weight gain will involve far less effort than trying to lose weight later on.

Try to stay as active as possible as you get older - exercise is still a major factor in a healthy life, helping to alleviate the symptoms of arthritis and increased joint mobility. In fact, you should be more active during middle age to burn off the extra calories that your slower metabolism is not using.

Identifying your specific nutritional needs and adapting your food intake accordingly is a lifelong commitment.

If, for example, you become ill and are bedridden, the nutritional value of your food needs to be high, but your calorie intake requirements will be reduced as you are completely inactive. If you are short of time and find it difficult to include exercise or activity in your day, a similar adjustment should be made. Conversely, it is important to maintain a healthy weight and not let your weight fall too low as you age - evidence suggests that fractures associated with osteoporosis are more likely among thinner people.

SUMMARY

There is no denying that the body undergoes natural changes as we age, and not for the better. Here's a summary:

- We get fatter
- Allergies become more of an issue
- Plaque builds up on our arteries
- We sweat less
- We reduce muscle mass
- The brain shrinks
- Our teeth become less sensitive
- Our skin becomes thinner, less elastic and drier
- Our hair becomes less vibrant
- We get shorter

- The bladder becomes weaker
- Our heart activity slows down
- Our taste sensation is reduced
- Our hormonal activity changes
- Our bone density decreases
- We experience digestive system disorders

As we age, we need to adjust our nutritional habits in order to offset these changes. The essence of those changes is that we need to eat fewer calories but receive higher nutrient density.

In order to meet their nutrient needs while eating fewer calories, older people should focus on eating the following whole foods:

- Vegetables
- Fruits
- Lean Meats
- Fish

The most important nutrients that are needed as we age are Vitamin B12, Vitamin D, Calcium and Protein.

STRESS AND OUR GUTS

"Breath is the power behind all things. I breathe in and know that good things will happen"

— TAO PORCHON-LYNCH

S tress is something that we all live with. The change and uncertainty that we are faced with on a daily basis present us with unique physiological, psychological and physical challenges. Our body's response to those challenges is what we call stress. Its physical manifestations are increased heart rate, muscle tension, elevated blood pressure and either expansion or constriction of our lung capacity. These changes prepare us for what is called the 'fight or flight syndrome,' in which the body is on 'high alert' to respond to the crisis.

Not all stress is bad. A controlled level of stress primes us to perform at our best. It allows us to react quickly to danger or to give extra effort to a challenging situation, such as going into a job interview. However, ongoing stress can be detrimental to our health, our thinking ability and our ability to perform and recover from exercise.

Stress affects every part of the body. Adrenaline and cortisol are released by the nervous system, which causes increased levels of blood pressure, heart rate and glucose. Too many of these hormones flowing through our system can result in headaches, irritability and insomnia.

Stress causes the muscles of our body to become tense. This is a protective mechanism to stave off injury. However, muscle tension can result in aches and pains, tension headaches and muscular spasms. Our rate of breathing increases as we work to bring in more oxygen. This can cause shortness of breath and hyperventilation. Stress will also cause the heart to beat faster in order to transport oxygen and nutrients to the muscles and organs of the body.

Stress also affects the way that we digest food. As a result, an inordinate amount of stress can lead to both diarrhea and constipation. Cloudy thinking, mental confusion and rash decision-making may also result from too much stress. It can cause us to act in ways that are out of character with our normal behavior. We may become sharp with others, make cutting remarks or fail to follow through on our responsibilities.

Stress can also lead to weight gain. Researchers have identified cortisol as the primary culprit in stress-related weight gain. They have also found that weight gain from cortisol primarily accumulates around the waistline!

STRESS AND AGING

Recent research indicates that the most stressful years in our lives are between the ages of 40 and 54. One study revealed that meeting financial obligations was a greater concern for people in this age group than at any other stage of life. A quarter of people over the age of 40 were also going through the stress of a relationship break up. Other major stressors for people in the 40-54 age group were the financial pressures of raising children and putting them through tertiary education, along with trying to prepare a nest egg for retirement.

Health problems related to aging were also found to be contributors to stress in this age group.

THE EFFECT OF STRESS ON YOUR GUT

Your body is home to around a hundred trillion microorganisms, each of which plays a vital role in the way your body looks and feels. Within your stomach lies an intricate complex of viruses, bacteria and fungi that are collectively referred to as your gut microbiome. It's also known as the Garden of Life. Just like any garden, your gut microbiome prospers when you look after it and deteriorates when you neglect it.

Since 2007, the Human Microbiome Project, a US National Institute of Health (NIH) research initiative, has examined the gut microbiome. In the process, more than a thousand species of microbes have been identified. The researchers have also identified the key jobs of your gut bacteria:

- It breaks down complex carbs
- It produces compounds such as vitamins B12, K, B3 and B6
- It produces short-chain fatty acids
- It strengthens the immune system
- It helps to detoxify the body
- It helps to protect the body from pathogens

- It modulates the nervous system

This is not an exhaustive list, but it is enough to give us an idea of the vital role the gut microbiome plays in orchestrating overall wellness. If you allow it to get out of sync, you will gain weight, opening yourself up to such complications as irritable bowel syndrome, heart disease and inflammatory bowel disease (IBD).

Recent research has shown your gut flora plays an essential role in weight control. It has been revealed that your gut microbes send fullness signals to your brain to tell it when to stop eating. In addition, the gut microbiome influences the vital balance between blood glucose and insulin levels. Your gut flora also controls your rate of metabolism.

All three of these factors – appetite control, blood glucose and insulin regulation and metabolism rate – are vital to weight control.

A large body of research makes it clear that stress has a major impact on gut health. The following gut issues have been directly linked to stress . . .

Inflammatory Bowel Disease (IBD)

A 2005 study that was published in *Gut* magazine concluded that chronic stress could increase the risk of relapse for people who suffered from IBDs such as

Crohn's Disease and ulcerative colitis. The researchers identified a number of mechanisms by which stress impacts both systemic and gastrointestinal immune and inflammatory responses.

Irritable Bowel Syndrome (IBS)

A study that involved more than 600 people found that the ability to handle stress was a key indicator as to whether patients whose gastroenteritis caused campylobacter went on to develop IBS.

Gastroesophageal Reflux Disease

One study found that, even though there was no indication that increased stress increases the frequency of acid reflux, stress does lead to an increased perception of acid reflux severity.

Peptic Ulcer Disease

While researchers no longer believe that Helicobacter Pylori (H. pylori) is directly caused by chronic stress, there is evidence that stress leads to mucosal lining inflammation, which allows gastric juices to irritate the lining of the stomach.

HOW STRESS AFFECTS THE DIGESTIVE SYSTEM

If you've ever had to give a speech, you probably already know that stress affects your stomach. What we commonly refer to as butterflies in the stomach is a physical manifestation of this phenomenon. It occurs because the brain and the gut are in constant communication. Your gut contains around 500 billion neurons which are collectively known as the enteric nervous system. These are partly controlled by the central nervous system in the brain.

The enteric nervous system is located in the gastrointestinal lining that runs from the esophagus to the rectum. It regulates the following processes:

- Swallowing
- Releasing enzymes that break down food
- Categorizing ingested nutrients as either food or waste products

When we are under stress, each of these processes is negatively impacted. Specifically, stress may cause the esophagus to spasm, increase acid build-up in the stomach, cause a nauseous feeling and lead to diarrhea or constipation.

HOW YOUR GUT BACTERIA GET OUT OF BALANCE

Let's start by considering where gut bacteria come from.

When you were in your mother's womb, you had a sterile environment within your intestines. The microbiome that you begin life with is inherited from her. It is transferred during the time you pass through the birth canal, as well as when you are breastfed.

Apart from the gut, the female vagina is home to a large population of gut flora. Some of this vaginal fluid is swallowed by the emerging baby. These are the first of the trillions of gut flora that colonize your intestines.

Breast milk contains bifidobacteria, which is an important probiotic. It also boosts the development of biofilms that line the gastrointestinal tract.

Some fascinating research has highlighted just how critical this formative gut flora is to lifelong weight control. A 2013 study by Azad et al showed that children who were born by C-section have much lower levels of healthy bacteria in their gut. This makes them more susceptible to serious illnesses, including allergies, asthma, inflammatory bowel syndrome, celiac disease and Type 1 Diabetes. They also found that babies who were born by C-section are at a higher risk for developing obesity.

A really interesting extra fact to come out of this study (and others like it) is that the microbial imbalances that begin at birth can last for up to 7 years.

Obviously, you had no control over what happened back then. But there are a number of other factors that contribute to the state of your gut's bacteria. The most influential one is nutrition.

Everything we eat is digested and metabolized by the flora in our gut. It is obvious, then, that your gut flora is operating optimally. That means that it has to be fed the right way.

So, what happens to your gut microbiome when you consume the typical American diet?

Foods that are high in processed carbohydrates, sugar, trans fats and artificial additives are, not surprisingly, bad news for your gut. The end result is that they will reduce the overall biodiversity of your gut flora. As reported in the journal *Future Microbiology,* an adjustment in the biodiversity of your gut microbiome leads to fat gain.

There are other factors that influence the state of health of your gut flora. Antibiotics are major bad news for your intestines. And yet, we have become a nation of prescription drug addicts. And we've turned our children into antibiotic dependents as well.

Mirroring the alarming increase in childhood drug dependency has been a considerable increase in the rate of childhood obesity. The connection is plain to see. In fact, a study by Bailey, LC, et al., which was published in the journal *JAMA Pediatrics* in 2014, revealed that youngsters who were given a broad spectrum of antibiotics prior to the age of two were far more likely to become obese during childhood.

Our environment is another big influencer on our gut bacteria. Species of flora come into the body when we're rolling around in the playground, kissing the dog, or even swallowing dirt.

As you are no doubt well aware, the mollycoddling nature of modern society has transformed the environmental influencers on our children. They don't play in the dirt anymore. We've become so bacteria phobic that our children are not being exposed to the natural influencers that can help to shape healthy gut bacteria.

Studies have shown children who are brought up on farms, where they are interacting with farm animals and getting back to nature, have a healthier balance of gut flora. As a result, they get sick less often and are less prone to obesity.

So, the over-sterilized, cotton wool environment that has been thrust upon us – and that we have, in turn, thrust upon our children – has not made a healthier society at all. It has, in fact, done the opposite . . .

It has set the stage for an epidemic of ill health and obesity.

THE MOOD / FOOD CONNECTION

Your food and your mood are directly related to one another. Yet, the vast majority of people are oblivious to this vital connection. They become obsessed with treating the symptoms of negative moods and miss out on the underlying causes. Often that cause is tied up with what you are putting down your throat.

The degradation of soil over the last fifty years has dramatically impacted the nutrient content of foods. In fact, it would take six apples for you to get the same nutritional value of just one apple from fifty years ago. On the African continent, the soil is nowhere as depleted as America. As a result, their fruits and vegetables are far more nutrient-dense. The result is that people who live over there generally have better teeth and bone structure.

One of the most important minerals for the body is potassium. It acts as a physiological tranquilizer, in effect calming the nervous system down. Bananas are well known for containing potassium. A single banana will provide 400 milligrams of potassium. However, we need 4700 milligrams of potassium per day just to meet our minimum daily requirement. That equates to 7-10 servings of vegetables per day.

You need potassium for two key reasons:

- To calm down your heart rate
- To maintain stable blood sugar levels

The B Vitamins are also very important for mood regulation. When you are feeling stressed, you quickly use up the B vitamins. This causes you to become more anxious and nervous. The most important B vitamin, and the one that gets exhausted first when you are stressed, is Vitamin B1. The best source of Vitamin B replacement is nutritional yeast. This can be picked up from your local health food store. Add a teaspoon to your yogurt or protein shake every day. It will help to calm you down as well as assisting you to get a good night's sleep.

Calcium is another key mineral for mood regulation. It helps to calm down and relax when you are in a stressed state. Stress causes calcium to pass right through the body without getting adequately absorbed. If you decide to supplement with a calcium product, do not use one that is derived from calcium carbonate. Instead, go for a supplement that is derived from calcium citrate, cheese or plain yogurt.

Omega-3 fatty acids are vital for proper brain functioning. You should supplement with high-quality fish oil, taking in 1000 mg per day.

Iodine is one more important mineral for mood elevation. Iodine supports the thyroid, which assists with the cognitive functioning of the brain. The best source of iodine is from sea kelp.

Regulating Blood Sugar

The amount of sugar in your blood has a direct effect on your mood. If your blood sugar level is too high, you are going to experience brain fog, typified by memory loss and impaired cognition. When the level is too low, you will become moody and irritable.

The biggest influencer on blood sugar levels is your consumption of simple carbohydrates. By switching around some of your basic eating habits, you can make considerable improvements in your blood sugar stability and, as a result, your mood.

Most people have been eating a carb-based breakfast their whole lives. It is either built around cereal or toast. This surges sugar into your body first thing in the morning, causing your blood sugar level to go up and resulting in a less than optimal cognitive functioning. The body's response to this high level of blood sugar is to release more insulin from the pancreas in order to clear the blood out. This leads to overcompensation and suddenly, you do not have enough sugar in the blood. Now you become moody and, around mid-morning hungry for more carbs to get your blood sugar levels back up. When you do, the whole vicious cycle repeats itself.

Simply by switching from a carb-based to a protein-based breakfast, you avoid all of these problems. Make eggs a staple of your breakfast menu and you'll be taking in close to 20 grams of high-grade protein to support lean muscle growth throughout the day (an average egg contains about 6 grams of protein. And you needn't worry about the cholesterol in the yolks. Scientists have recently shown that there are no issues with up to eating 2-3 eggs per day.

You should also consider having a whey-based protein shake as a breakfast alternative. Look for a low-carb protein mix that contains whey isolate protein, as it will digest faster than other forms. A protein-based breakfast will help to stabilize your blood sugar levels right throughout the remainder of the day. Avoiding sugar is the most important thing you can do to improve your mood.

Hormones and Your Mood

Hormones have a huge influence on your brain, and therefore your mood. Serotonin is a pleasure hormone that makes you feel good. It acts as a neurotransmitter that sends messages to your brain. You can thus build up your serotonin levels through your diet. To do so, you can increase your consumption of foods that contain tryptophan, the amino acid which is the building block of serotonin.

The following ten foods are all high in tryptophan:

- Free-range turkey
- Flaxseed
- Buckwheat
- Wild fish
- Whey protein
- Bananas
- Eggs
- Sour cherries
- Free-range beef
- Dark chocolate

Cortisol is the stress hormone. It leads to anxiety and constant worry, where your mind is going at a hundred miles an hour thinking about negative things. Exercising and maintaining a clean diet that is free of junk food and simple carbs are two of the best strategies for keeping your cortisol levels down.

The following foods will help you to control your cortisol levels:

- Coldwater fish
- Walnuts
- Swiss Chard
- Eggs
- Dark chocolate
- Greek Yogurt
- Citrus Fruit
- Pumpkin seeds
- Spinach

Food and beverages to avoid to control cortisol . . .

- Alcohol
- Caffeine
- Low fiber carbohydrates
- Flavored yogurt
- Fruit juice
- Trans fats

STRESS & WEIGHT GAIN

Stress not only makes us cranky, irritable and frazzled; it also makes us fatter. Recent research has shown that stress-induced cortisol release leads to fat gain. Specifically, cortisol fat gain tends to collect around the middle of the body. A 2011 study found that women with greater abdominal fat had more negative moods and higher levels of life stress. The lead researcher, Elissa S. Epel, Ph.D., concluded that 'greater exposure to life stress or psychological vulnerability to stress may explain their enhanced cortisol reactivity. In turn, their cortisol exposure may have led them to accumulate greater abdominal fat.'

Conversely, when cortisol levels are lowered, abdominal fat levels come down. In another study, researchers from the University of California at San Francisco randomly assigned chronically stressed overweight and obese women to nine weekly sessions (lasting two and a half hours each) of mindfulness training and practice, where they learned stress reduction and awareness techniques. Additionally, the women in the mindfulness group were asked to meditate for thirty minutes a day. The control group received no mindfulness training. Although no diets were prescribed, both groups did attend one session about the basics of healthy eating and exercise.

Then, the researchers measured the participants' psychological stress, fat, deep abdominal fat, weight, and cortisol levels before and after the four-month study. The link they found was clear: when women's cortisol levels went down, so did their abdominal fat levels. Further, those with the most significant reductions in cortisol had the greatest reductions in abdominal fat.

The link between stress-induced cortisol levels and abdominal fat gain couldn't be clearer. Incorporating the mindful breathing technique can help you control stress and bring down your cortisol level.

STRESS & THINKING ABILITY

One of the most immediate effects of stress is to impact our ability to think clearly. Cortisol, the same hormone that causes abdominal weight gain, will alter the structure and function of the brain. Excess levels of cortisol cause overproduction of a neurotransmitter called glutamate. Too much glutamate is not good; in fact, it becomes a neurotoxin which causes free radical activity that can actually kill brain cells.

One of the most immediate stress-related cognitive effects is forgetfulness. Stress causes electrical signals in the brain, which weaken the memory. At the same time, the parts of the brain associated with emotion are enhanced. That makes us more likely to make rash decisions based upon emotion and less likely to follow through on our healthy lifestyle choices. In other words, when you're stressed, you are more likely to make the decision to ditch your workout and reach for a cookie instead!

STRESS' IMPACT ON METABOLISM

Have you ever noticed that your body doesn't seem to digest food very well when you're overly stressed? It's no coincidence. Stress and the stomach are unavoidably linked. That's because the portion of the brain that activates stress deactivates digestion. A part of the central nervous system called the autonomic nervous system (ANS) turns on the gastric processes in the stomach that allow us to digest food. The ANS also tells the stomach when to switch off. When our body switches into fight or flight mode, it switches off digestion. As a result, we experience gastric problems.

Cortisol is one of the key drivers that puts us into fight or flight mode. This hormone speeds up the breakdown of glucose and fat to provide the body with the energy required to respond to the emergency situation that it perceives when we are under stress. This results in an increased metabolism.

TOP 10 WAYS TO DEAL WITH STRESS

We can't avoid stress. It is the body's inbuilt device to help us to cope with what life throws at us. From the moment we crawl out of bed until the time we return to the covers, it is a constant that we have to contend with. So, removing stress from our lives is an unrealistic goal.

What we can do is to learn to better manage the stress that we encounter. For most people, stress is brought about when the events in their life are uncontrollable or unpredictable. Many people, in fact, define stress as being the time when they feel as if they have no control over their lives. Research has shown that when people learn to relinquish control over every aspect of their life, they feel less stressed.

Here are ten scientifically proven ways to more meaningfully manage your stress.

Stress Buster #1: Learn to Breathe

Learning to breathe correctly is the most fundamental thing you can do to reduce your stress levels and improve your overall wellbeing. Your basic life processes, such as your heartbeat and respiration, are controlled by your autonomic nervous system. For a long time, it was believed that we had no conscious control over its operation.

We now know that many aspects of the autonomic nervous system can be controlled by the individual. The way we control them is by breathing from the belly. The simplest and most direct form of stress management is to move from a shallow, stressed state of breathing into deep, belly breathing.

In learning to breathe again, you will be consciously thinking about your breathing - perhaps for the first time in your life. After a while, though, you'll no longer have to think about it. Deep breathing will become habitual. Until then, however, you will need to consciously make an effort to breathe correctly. You won't be breathing properly with every breath straight away and you shouldn't expect to.

Start by taking in deep breaths for 20 seconds every hour. Slowly increase until you are doing it for a minute at a time. After a week, you'll be up to 5 or 6 minutes every hour. At the end of 3 months, the old ineffective way of getting oxygen into your system will be a thing of the past. Your body will no longer be sputtering down the road on half a cylinder - you'll be cruising along on all 4 cylinders, with the hood down and the wind blowing through your hair!

How to Do It

Stand or sit comfortably. Now, take in a long, deep breath through your nose until the lungs are completely full and your chest is inflated. Hold this breath for 5 full seconds. Now, allow the breath to slowly leave your body. Be thinking about expanding and compressing the diaphragm as if it were an accordion on every inward and outward breath.

The Power of Nasal Breathing

Learning to breathe through your nose will make you a far more effective in-taker of oxygen. When you inhale through the nose, you will be taking the air more deeply into your diaphragm. Try it right now and you will be able to feel your diaphragm expanding. This expansion puts downward pressure on your abdomen. This has the flow-on effect of pushing air into the lungs and enhancing the circulation of blood and nutrients. This form of breathing is also more relaxing than mouth breathing.

Test Yourself: Breathe 100

Take in 100 nasal breaths in a row. Exhale through your mouth each time. Next, focus on breathing in with just your right nostril—breathe out through your left. After 100 breaths, swap sides. As a final nasal challenge, breathe in 100 times, holding for 10 seconds after each breath.

Sub-10: Your Breathing Goal

When you are breathing optimally, you will be taking in no more than 10 breaths a minute, ideally just seven or eight. Your goal is to achieve as many sub-10 breath minutes as possible in your day.

Breathing Exercise

The breathing method just outlined will allow you to dramatically improve the amount of oxygen that comes into your body. That's great moving forward. However, you still have to contend with a whole lifetime of ineffective breathing. The following breathing exercise will allow you to strengthen and maintain power in your lungs.

Do this first thing in the morning upon waking and again in the mid-afternoon (it will provide a caffeine-free way of overcoming the 3 o'clock slump!).

Step One: Get comfortable, either standing or sitting.
Step Two: Breathe in through the nose for 5 seconds. Feel your stomach pushing out as the energy-giving oxygen fills your lungs.
Step Three: Hold for 20 seconds. Feel the oxygen

circulating around your body as it gives life to your trillions of cells.

Step Four: Repeat this process four more times.

When performing lung exercises, it is important to focus on inflating the lungs upward and outward rather than downward. Imagine that the intake of oxygen is about to lift you up and carry you skyward.

The Pay Off

Learning to breathe correctly will be frustrating and annoying to start with. But remember back to when you began to learn to ride a bike? That was frustrating. It was annoying. And it was probably painful. But you persevered. If you had given up, you probably wouldn't be whizzing around in a car today. Same thing with learning to breathe. In fact, there are at least 14 direct benefits that come with deep breathing:

- Enhanced toxin release
- Enhanced tension release
- Better clarity and relaxation
- Relieves emotional pressure
- Eases physical pain
- Increases muscle mass
- Strengthens immune system
- Enhances digestion of food

- Enhances nervous system functioning
- Strengthens the lungs
- Helps burn fat
- Boosts energy levels
- Enhances cellular regeneration
- Makes you happier

Stress Buster #2: Learn to Appreciate

Too often, we take life for granted. Yet, learning to appreciate what we have by seeing the good and the value in what we have right now is a key stress reducer.

It is very easy to fix our attention on all the things that are going wrong in our lives. It takes real effort for us to see the good, even though it's right in front of our faces. In fact, the very process of slowing down in order to 'smell the roses' is difficult for most people. The ironic thing is that it is this inability to slow down and appreciate the everyday little things that is a key stress contributor.

When you train your mind to think about the good things that you have, despite the negative curveballs that come your way, you can actually reverse the stress response.

Here is how you can purposefully implement the appreciation strategy:

When you wake up in the morning, mentally review the things you need to do in the day and include on that list two things that you are grateful for.

When you feel stress coming on, take two deep belly breaths. When you inhale for the third breath, let your mind focus on someone you love, a place you enjoy being at, or an act of kindness someone has done for you.

Throughout your day, regularly focus on someone you love, a place you enjoy being at, or an act of kindness someone has done for you for up to 30 seconds at a time.

Stress Buster #3: Slow Down

Life is hectic. Everybody is in such a hurry to get from Point A to Point B and to move from one thing to the next. We have appallingly short attention spans and we have lost the ability to be patient and wait. All of those things are bound to bring on stress.

The simple act of slowing down is a fundamental skill that will make your life more relaxed. It is only when we learn to slow down that we truly get to appreciate the beauty of the lives that we live. Slowing down is not difficult, but making it a practice in your life can be. To succeed you need to work at it.

Start by taking notice of what you eat. Take the time to taste and savor your food. This eating with attentive care will help you to make smarter food choices and avoid weight gain.

You don't have to slow down all day long, but you should have an OFF switch that allows you to slow down when you want to. Slowing down will put less strain on your body and give you more energy as you go about your daily activities.

To instigate the slowing down process, simply tell yourself that you have all the time in the world. As you slow down, become totally absorbed in and focused on what you are doing. Doing so will not only reduce stress – it will make you a much better person to be around!

Stress Buster #4: Relax Your Muscles

When we get stressed, our muscles become tense. In fact, our bodies can become so used to this bunched-up feeling of tension that we are no longer able to relax, even when we aren't stressed. It is possible, however, to train the body to react in a relaxed manner to a stressful situation.

Stress brings about a natural tightness of muscle and restricted flow of blood to the hands and the feet. Tense muscles feel heavy, whereas relaxed muscles feel light. The interesting thing is that our muscles are the most relaxed immediately after they have been tensed.

Consciously tensing and relaxing is a skill that you can develop in order to alleviate stress. You can even do this while driving the car. Grip the steering wheel tightly and then relax your grip. You'll immediately feel how relaxed the muscles in your arms feel.

Here's how to apply this life skill . . .

Before you go to bed, exercise, sitting at your desk or are stuck in traffic, take two slow, deep belly breaths.
On the third inhalation, tighten your right arm from the shoulder to the hand.
How this position for three seconds.
As you exhale, relax the arm entirely and let it drop.
Repeat with the other arm.

Stress Buster #5: Visualize Success

Visualizing success involves removing from your mind the negative images of failure that you have and replacing them with positive images of success. When you visualize success, your body will immediately relax and the body calms itself. In contrast, the practice that most people have of constantly feeding themselves negativity leads to stress.

To make success visualization work for you, think about an area of your life in which you are not successful. Now take three slow, deep belly breaths. Now build up an image of yourself succeeding at that activity. Next, describe to yourself what the image showed you about how to be successful at the activity. Ask yourself how success was different from the things you usually do. Now plan ways to implement that knowledge into your future performance.

Practice this process at least three times for every area of your life that you want to find more success in.

Stress Buster #6: Appreciate Yourself

The majority of people out there see a glass as being half empty, especially when that glass is themselves. They fixate on their failings without giving any credit to themselves for their good points. Learning to appreciate yourself will lead to an immediate reduction in stress along with greater self-contentment.

Learning to appreciate yourself essentially comes back to self-talk. The vast majority of our self-talk is negative. We tell ourselves that we are a failure, that we are not as good, not as attractive or not as smart. Life coaching guru Zig Ziglar referred to this as 'stinkin' thinkin'.

It is your job to banish 'stinkin' thinkin' from your life. When a negative thought enters your mind, quash it and replace it with a positive one. Every day, think of at least one thing that you did that was helpful or something that you were good at.

Be confident in the person that you are. Know your identity and values and be proud of them. If they are out of step with the mainstream, don't feel the need to apologize for them. Appreciate yourself, be proud and confident, and you will project an aura of confidence that will be attractive to others.

Stress Buster #7: Change Behaviors

You've probably heard of the quote which is most often attributed to Albert Einstein that says that 'the definition of insanity is doing the same thing over and over and expecting a different result.' Often the behaviors that cause stress are things that we repeat over and over again. Changing those behaviors is a key to stress relief.

To make this stress buster a success, you need to identify the things that aren't working in your life and stop doing them. Then, implement a new strategy that may bring a better result.

Often, the thing that is causing us frustration is not knowing how to solve our problems. As a result, we just flip back to the old, familiar, unsuccessful ways. Having the patience to seek out and implement a better way will go a long way to relieving your stress.

Stress Buster #8: Learn to Say No

Often our stress is due to the fact that we cannot say no. As a result, we accept too much responsibility. Remember that the world won't end if you don't accept every request that comes your way.

Many people find it difficult to be assertive in certain situations and with certain people. But when you are able to, you can completely avoid many potentially stressful situations. When we don't clearly state our opinion, we can end up in an anxious position. Psychiatrists refer to this as 'suppression' and it can result in low self-esteem and severe depression.

To effectively use this skill, you need to be able to:

- Know when saying no is appropriate (whenever you have a choice)
- Understand the difference between being assertive, being non-assertive and being aggressive
- Practice saying no in simple, non-threatening

situations initially before moving on to more challenging situations.

Stress Buster #9: Accept the Unchangeable

When we learn to make a distinction between the changeable and the unchangeable, we can come to peace with the fact that we cannot always be in control. The things we cannot change we should accept. It is encapsulated in what has come to be known as the Serenity Prayer:

Grant me the serenity to accept the things I cannot change,
The courage to change the things I can,
And the wisdom to know the difference.

The key message here is to make things better when you can and to also understand the times when you don't have the power to change a situation. And if you can't change it, it is illogical to stress out about it. Accept it and move on.

If you are stuck in traffic and are late for an appointment, accepting the unchangeable will allow you to be at peace with the situation. Rather than stressing out, you will simply accept the fact that you will be late, turn on the radio and enjoy the music.

Stress Buster #10: Exercise

You know that exercise is a great way to relieve stress. You've probably even heard of the feel-good hormones known as endorphins which lift your mood and generally make you feel good about life.

Regular exercise buys into many of the stress busters that we have already considered. It allows you to carve out of the time of the day that is just for you and also the time when you are able to work on maintaining and improving yourself. This allows you to slow down, build your self-esteem and develop your appreciation for yourself. Studies show that regular cardiovascular exercise significantly improves mental alertness and concentration, reduces stress and improves overall physical and mental wellbeing

The key to exercise success is regularity. Find an activity that you genuinely enjoy and perform it an average of thirty minutes per day. Doing so will enable you to improve your fitness level and lose weight as you get a handle on your stress level.

SUMMARY

Stress is an unavoidable part of all of our lives, but recent research indicates that it affects people aged between 40-54 more than any other age group. A raft of research has shown that stress has a direct impact on our physical health, especially digestion and gut health. The best nutrients to reduce stress are:

- Potassium
- B Vitamins
- Calcium
- Omega-3 Fatty Acids
- Iodine

Reducing your sugar intake will significantly reduce your stress levels. One way you can do this is to switch from a carb-based to a protein-based breakfast. You should also increase your concentration of foods that contain tryptophan as well as those that control your cortisol levels.

Here are 10 foods to include in your diet to help reduce your stress levels:

- Spinach
- Cold water fish
- Swiss Chard
- Cheese
- Plain Yogurt
- Eggs
- Dark Chocolate
- Citrus Fruits

- Walnuts
- Pumpkin seeds

Here are 10 things you can do to keep your stress levels at bay:

- Practice deep nasal breathing
- Learn to appreciate what you have
- Slow down
- Relax your muscles
- Visualize success
- Appreciate yourself
- Change behaviors
- Learn to say no
- Accept the unchangeable
- Exercise

WHY DIETS DON'T WORK FOR MOST PEOPLE

"Guilt has no place when it comes to eating"

— EVELYN TRIBOLE

L osing weight is big business. The diet industry is booming with the old standbys like Jenny Craig and Weight Watchers going from strength to strength even as new diets seem to emerge every other day. The integration of diet culture with the social media obsession on physical appearance has fueled the weight loss obsession even further. As a result, many people are still falling into the diet trap despite the overwhelming evidence that diets don't work for most people.

In this chapter, we get to the truth about dieting. You'll discover what really happens to your body when you go on – and off – a diet, how it affects not only your body composition but your overall long-term health, and why diets will never lead to long-term weight loss success. You will also realize that if you've tried and failed on diets in the past, it's not your fault – it's simply further proof that the diet model is fundamentally flawed.

First though, let's consider why diets are still so wildly popular, despite the undeniable evidence that they don't really work.

Why Are Diets So Popular

According to the US Federal Trade Commission, the Diet Industry is the only profitable industry in the world with a 98% failure rate. Think about that for a moment – for every hundred people who go on a diet, only two of them achieve their goal, which is long-term weight loss. Imagine if you were selling a product that failed 98 percent of users. You'd soon be out of business. Yet, the diet industry just keeps going from strength to strength!

How can this be?

A big part of the answer lies in our society's obsession with the thin body. Even in these 'woke' times, Western culture continues to hold up the fat-free body as the physical ideal. It's interesting to note that this is not the case in other parts of the world. Many African tribes, for example, consider excess body fat, especially in females, to be an attractive quality. Not only is it seen as sexy, but it is also an indicator of wealth and status.

In the western world, just the opposite view pervades. Fat is the enemy. And dieting remains the most popular way to defeat it. Here are the top five reasons why we continue to fall into the diet trap.

Diets are Sold as the Solution to Our Problems

The power of the media to influence is stronger than most people realize. From our formative years, we are bombarded with images and messages convincing us that we need to torch fat from our bodies. As a result, many of us link the loss of fat with the achievement of our goals. We tell ourselves that we'll be able to advance in our career when we achieve our goal weight or that we'll be able to start dating online when we get rid of 20 pounds. This provides a very powerful emotional driver to do whatever we have to get the weight off. And when our emotions take over, any intellectual knowledge that dieting isn't going to provide the solution we're looking for will get squashed and we'll allow ourselves to be overtaken by the next and latest glamour fad diet.

The Short-Term Fix Effect

When people do lose weight on a diet, they are celebrated as having achieved something really wonderful. They post before and after pics on Instagram, people comment on their new look and they feel great about themselves. All of that is great. The problem is that 98 percent of people will not only put the weight back on but actually end up heavier than they were before they started the diet.

In effect, going on a diet is a bit like getting a short-term high only to suffer a long-term crash. Even if you know the crash is coming, the lure of the high is very hard to resist!

The Personal Challenge Effect

We all love a challenge. And the diet industry presents us with the opportunity to rely on our willpower and discipline to challenge ourselves in order to conquer our bodies. When people go on diets, they love to talk about it with their peers. Often, they pair up with a friend and it becomes part of a social bonding process. Social media is used as a platform to provide support and reinforcement. The diet, in effect, is part of the relationship.

Diet challenges are especially attractive. These are increasingly being pushed online with the social aspect and the prospect of winning and becoming a social media' star' drawing in many people.

Diets Put You on Auto-Pilot

Diets provide a paint-by-numbers approach to weight loss. So long as we buy the book or sign up to the program, we don't have to think about what we should eat and when. We simply follow the template. Many people find that to be an extremely attractive proposition.

Celebrity Endorsements

Celebrities have been making money from diet endorsements for a long time. They continue to do so because their endorsements carry a lot of weight (no pun intended). Social media platforms have allowed celebrities to share more of their lives with their fans than ever. As a result, we get to see them following a diet as they go through their normal routine. Of course, they are really nothing more than the social media equivalent of product placement ads but they can make a big impression on someone who idolizes that celebrity.

WHY DIETS DON'T WORK

So far in this chapter, I've made it clear that diets are not the solution if you are after long-term weight loss. Let's now back up that assertion. Here are a half dozen reasons why you should never go on a diet.

Your Metabolism is Negatively Affected

Most people throw around the word metabolism without really knowing what it is. We've been conditioned to thinking that we've either got a fast or slow metabolism, with most of us convincing ourselves that we've got an extremely slow one – otherwise, we'd be able to lose weight, right?

The truth is that your metabolism – the rate at which all of the chemical reactions that occur within your body in order to keep you alive – is constantly fluctuating.

The metabolism was created to deal with the conditions that our original ancestors faced. Back then, finding food took a great deal of energy. In fact, it was likely that a person would go for a lengthy period of time without any food at all. The metabolism was designed in such a way that, when we ate less, it slowed down. This was a natural starvation response to preserve calories so that we had enough energy to carry us through.

Today, of course, we hardly ever find ourselves in a real life or death starvation situation. Yet, the metabolism works the same as it did back then. When we *choose* to eat less, such as when we go on a restricted-calorie diet, the metabolism will gradually slow down. That means that we will be burning energy more slowly.

As a result of this natural 'starvation response' the body actually works against dieting. It is doing so in order to prepare you for a coming famine, with the effect that you will actually store fat more readily. Your body doesn't know that you are consciously choosing to cut back on calories. It responds as if you were in an emergency situation to prevent you from starving. Hormonal changes take place to allow you to hoard body fat as stored energy just the same way a bear does in preparation for hibernation over the winter.

Psychological Defeatism

When we go on a diet, we become obsessed with food. It's the classic pink elephant scenario. If you are told not to think about a pink elephant, what will constantly pop into your head over the next five minutes?

You got it . . . images of pink elephants!

Same thing with food. If you are told not to eat certain foods for a long period of time, you will particularly think about the foods that have been forbidden to you. This makes the task of sticking to the diet that much harder.

Another thing that happens when we restrict our eating is that we get more stressed. A 2010 study out of Los Angeles proved for the first time that diets are stressful and lead to the release of the cortisol hormone. This, in turn, leads to the temptation to binge eat and keeps you awake at night, inhibiting the release of the hunger or satiety hormones ghrelin and leptin. In these ways, the stress will also make you fatter.

Research shows that the brain responds differently to food when you are dieting. It becomes far more tuned in to food. As a result, you will pick up flavors and aromas more readily. When you come in contact with appetizing food, your taste buds will salivate faster than when you are not dieting. It has even been shown that the prefrontal cortex, which is the portion of the brain that controls temptation, is less active when you are dieting.

Weight Loss Obsession

A major problem with low-calorie diets is that they do not differentiate between weight loss and fat loss. You should never be interested in losing pure weight. Being obsessed with bringing your weight down on the scale is misguided – pure and simple.

The bathroom scale cannot differentiate between muscle and fat. Nor can it tell if you are losing water or vital minerals. All it can tell you is that your overall body weight has gone down. That, in itself, is a useless piece of information.

You never want to lose muscle. Yet, on most calorie-restricted diets, that is exactly what you are losing. Muscle weighs five times more than fat. So, when a person's body goes into starvation response because they have severely cut back their caloric intake, the body turns to its muscle stores and starts to catabolize itself.

When you step on the scale, you feel elated. The scale has come down. But what have you actually done to your body? You have robbed it of its body shaping, firming, strength-enhancing muscle mass. Meanwhile, most of your fat is still there, where it's always been.

You can be on a calorie-reduced diet and still be incredibly unhealthy. Likewise, you can actually increase your calories by eating more nutritionally rich food whilst exercising regularly and you can actually lose fat and gain muscle. Just think how much food professional athletes put away on a daily basis. In 2014, Olympic wrestling gold medal winner Kurt Angle revealed that he would have around 7 meals per day, eating every two hours. He was of course, on an elite training regime, but he was in incredible shape and far from being considered fat.

Reduced calorie diets will also squeeze water weight from your body, especially in the initial stages. We've already discussed the vital importance of water in the body, so you know that is not a good thing. Yet, again, it fools people into thinking that they are losing body fat.

Research Show It Doesn't Work for Most of Us

The conventional wisdom about losing weight hasn't changed for more than a hundred years. That thinking tells us that it is all about calories. If you consume calories in excess of those burned through metabolism and inactivity, you'll get fat. So, obviously, in order to lose that fat, you've got to eat fewer calories and exercise more.

The only problem is that millions of people have been doing just that – and actually getting fatter! There is also a mountain of both anecdotal and research-based evidence to show that this approach needs to not be looked at so simplistically. Let's take a look at an example of a calorie-reduced diet.

In one study published in the journal *Lancet* in 2009, participants with an average age of 36 and an average Body Mass Index (BMI) of 35 were put on a calorie-reduced diet (1,000 calories reduction) for a full 12 months. Half of them also exercised. After twelve months, the results were as follows:

Diet only group: 0.9 kg lost
Diet and exercise: 2.2 kg lost

Another 12-month study involved people with an average age of 42 who had an average BMI of 36.5. These people were put on a diet of between 1,200 and 1,500 calories per day. Half of them also did regular aerobic exercise, resistance exercise. Results were:

Diet only group: 4.6 kg lost
Diet and exercise: 5.2 kg lost

A third study had people with an average age of 45 and an average BMI of 36 put on a low-fat diet containing 800-1,000 calories per day. Again, half of them were given exercise in the form of brisk walking for 3 miles, 5 times per week. This lasted for two years. Results were:

Diet only group: 2.1 kg lost

Diet and exercise: 2.5 kg lost

Our final study involved men with an average age of 43 and an average BMI of 25.5. They followed a low-fat, high-carb diet for 12 months. Once more, some of the group added exercise, this time in the form of 30 minutes of aerobic exercise, 4-5 times per week. Results were:

Diet only group: No change in weight
Diet and exercise: 1.9 kg lost

Let's now take a look at a summary of those results . . .

Study	Length (months)	Weight change (kg) – diet only	Weight change (kg) – diet and exercise
1	12	-0.9	-2.2
2	12	-4.6	-5.2
3	24	-2.1	-2.5
4	12	0.0	-1.9
Average	-	-1.9	-2.95

So, what do we learn from these diet studies?

After an average of 12 months of hardcore dieting, the average weight loss was just 2 kg. Even when exercise was added to the equation, the average weight loss only went up to 3 kg. Keep in mind, too, that the people on these studies had an abundance of professional support and guidance. The bottom line is that traditional dieting methods, those based on caloric restriction, are in many cases, a fast track to failure.

FAD DIET DANGER SIGNS

From what we've considered so far in this chapter, it should be clear that fad diets are just another bad food habit that needs to be avoided. So, let's pause for a moment and consider just what a fad diet is.

The word diet has had its original meaning corrupted over the past 100 years. Originally your diet simply referred to what you ate. But now the word is used to describe a period of restricted eating where you cut back on calories and avoid certain types of food. A fad diet will often center around a specific type of food. Others severely restrict or cut out a food group like carbohydrates.

Here are the characteristics of a fad diet to look out for and avoid . . .

- The diet cuts out a macronutrient – any type of diet that severely restricts one of the food groups is bad news. Not only is it extremely difficult to sustain such a diet, but you will struggle to meet your body's fuel needs if you cut back too much on any macronutrient.

- They describe their diet as being 'easy' – losing weight the right way isn't easy. With all of the bad food choices that we are surrounded with, it requires consistency, discipline and self-control. Any diet that tells you otherwise is lying to you.
- The diet promises rapid weight loss – you can lose weight fast but you cannot lose fat fast. Slow and steady fat loss is the way to go.
- The diet requires that you follow strict rules that are unrealistic in the real world.
- The diet claims scientific backing but it is based on in-house research or anecdotal evidence.

Negative Effects of Fad Diets

Fads are not only ineffective. They can also be dangerous. Here are 10 negative effects that may result from going on a fad diet . . .

- Dehydration
- Overhydration
- Muscle loss
- Reduced bone density

- Lack of energy
- Headaches
- Low blood sugar
- Heart damage
- Nutritional deficiencies
- Constipation

What Happens When the Diet Ends?

By its definition, a fad diet comes to an end. So, what happens when that expiration date rolls around? For many dieters, the end of the diet is binge time. They compensate for all those weeks of restrictive eating by splurging out on the sugary, sweet foods they've been missing on. This binge eating is not just the result of a lack of willpower; the diet model itself actually drives it.

Diets create forbidden foods in the mind of the dieter. As we noted with the example of pink elephants, we can't help but obsess over these out-of-bounds foods. The brain is overstimulated to light up when these foods come on our radar. It's hardly surprising that when the diet is over and the restrictions are off, we go crazy and splurge on cakes, cookies and junk food.

When a dieter goes on a post-diet binge, they'll often justify it by telling themselves that it is a one-off – and that they deserve it. But it is hardly ever a one-off! In fact, it is part of a vicious cycle. Binge eating leads to shame and guilt, which causes one to jump onto another fad diet. When they come off the diet, they binge again and the process repeats. This cycle has been the pattern for millions of people for years.

WHAT ABOUT INTERMITTENT FASTING?

One of the most popular diets to emerge in recent years has been Intermittent Fasting. It is centered more around the timing of your eating than the actual foods that you eat. Intermittent fasting involves periods of fasting followed by an eating window. The fasting period could range from 12 hours to more than 40 hours. The most popular form of IF is the 16:8 diet, in which the dieter fasts for 16 hours of each 24-hour period and eats for the remaining 8 hours. Here is how it may look . . .

You stop eating at 7pm. You then fast until 11am the following morning. Then, between 11am and 7pm you eat your food.

So, how effective is Intermittent Fasting when it comes to long-term fat loss? A recent major study suggests that there is no evidence that time-restricted eating works as a weight-loss strategy. In the study, one group of people were put on an IF regimen of 8 hour feeding windows and 16 hour fasting periods each day. At the end of 12 weeks, they had lost an average of 2 pounds. Another group ate normally with similar foods at the same caloric intake for 12 weeks. They lost an average of 1.5 pounds. The researchers concluded that the difference was not statistically significant. The fasting group were also shown to lose more muscle mass over the period of the study than the control group.

There does, however, need to be more research on the effects of intermittent fasting for long-term weight loss. The research that currently exists, however, suggests that it may not be the panacea that many are proclaiming it to be.

SUMMARY

In this chapter, we have clearly established that dieting is not the solution to long-term weight loss. Despite having a 98 percent failure rate, however, they continue to be the weight loss option of choice for the majority of people as a result of . . .

- Media influence
- The short-term fix effect
- The solution to all our problems effect
- Their paint by numbers approach
- Celebrity endorsements

Yet, despite how popular fad diets are, the science of how the body works means that they can never be successful. When you go on a diet the following things occur . . .

- Your metabolism slows down
- Your body kicks into fight or flight mode
- Your cortisol levels increase
- Stress levels rise
- You fixate on forbidden foods
- You tend to lose muscle tissue, water and minerals over fat

Then when you go off the diet, there is a high likelihood that you will binge eat, which leads to rebound weight gain. In fact, research confirms that the vast majority of dieters end up fatter in the long run than before they started the diet.

The message is clear – if you are interested in long-term fat loss, steer clear of diets!

STEP TWO. CHANGING MINDSET

IDENTIFYING THE RULES & HABITS WE NOW LIVE BY

"You don't have to see the whole staircase, just take the first step"

— MARTIN LUTHER KING

I n the first section of this book, we have established that our eating habits are heavily influenced by our upbringing and our environment. But that doesn't mean that our nutritional future is predetermined. We all have the power within us to break free of the bad nutritional habits that have got us to where we are. The first step in that process is to identify the habits that have developed as subconscious eating rules in our own lives. By becoming mindful of what we are doing, we will be in a position to challenge and change it.

Want an example of how powerful mindfulness is when it comes to our eating habits? Like most people, you may have the habit of chowing down on potato chips while watching TV. But try eating a packet of potato chips while you're staring at your naked self in the mirror or, better yet, standing on the bathroom scales! Suddenly those chips won't be so appetizing. What's the difference? You're now mindfully aware of the consequences of your eating habit!

In this chapter, I'm going to challenge you to identify the eating habits that have become ingrained in your life over the years. To do this, you'll be presented with a number of interactive activities that will help you to become a mindful detective about your current eating habits.

To successfully identify and then overcome your unproductive eating habits, you need to go into this process without judgment. Now is not the time to condemn yourself or feel guilty about the bad eating habits you have developed. Rather than being judgmental, be curious. Curiosity opens you up to creativity, which is the spark that leads to positive change.

MINDFUL EATING

Most people go through life on automatic pilot. They perform their daily activities without any thought while their brain is consumed with something else. As a result, they miss the gift of the present while their mind is either regretting the past or worrying about the future. Mindfulness is the counter to living your life on automatic pilot. Although it is a relatively new concept in the consciousness of the western world, mindfulness has been around for a long time. In the 1960s, the famous missionary Mother Teresa summed up the whole essence of mindfulness with this simple statement . . .

"Be happy in the moment. That's enough. Each moment is all we need, not more."

The opposite of mindfulness is mindlessness. It involves doing what you have always done without thinking about it. When you live like that, you are not in control of your life. Mindfulness puts you back in the driver's seat, allowing you to live a purposeful life.

Here are 8 principles that form the basis of mindfulness:

- Be in the moment, slow down and think about what you are doing NOW
- Realize that you have the power to change
- Trust your gut instincts
- Attune your mind and body
- Become aware of your habits
- Be curious, not judgmental
- Take responsibility for your actions
- Maintain an open, flexible mind

Mindful eating applies the principles of mindfulness to your eating habits. It is all about being fully aware of your habits, cravings and behaviors regarding the nutrients that go into your body. When you eat mindfully, you are able to eat the foods that you want when you want to rather than being a slave to your habitual behaviors.

Many people find that mindful eating becomes a catalyst to taking control of other areas of their lives as well. As a result, they become more empowered, more connected and happier.

Here is a 6-step process that will help you to become a mindful eater . . .

Control What Comes into the House

Mindful eating begins at the supermarket. That is the source of most of the food that comes into your house. Start at the vegetable section and spend time exploring. Choose a wide range of vegetable types and colors. Look for veggies that are new to you and give them a try.

Shop on the outskirts of the store. Think about the nutritional impact of everything that goes into your trolley. If you allow yourself a treat food, do it mindfully, having planned it into your week. Be especially in the moment when you are at the checkout as that is where the most tempting sugar-laden snacks will be hanging out.

Don't Allow Yourself to Get Too Hungry

If you come to the dinner table with a ravenous appetite, there is a very high likelihood that you will stuff yourself so full of food that you'll end up feeling very uncomfortable. You won't be thinking about what you're eating or about your satiety cues.

You can avoid getting overly hungry between meals by eating a quality source of lean protein with each meal, spacing your meals about three hours apart and drinking plenty of water throughout the day.

Buy Smaller Plates

The diameter of the average dinner plate sold over the past 60 years has expanded right along with people's waistlines. In the 1950's that diameter was 9 inches, while today it is 13.5 inches. Most of us have been conditioned to cleaning up everything on our plate, even if we feel we've had enough. This leads to overeating and a daily caloric surplus, which leads to fat storage.

The simple remedy is to buy smaller dinner plates. Reduce down to 9 inches and your waistline will also come down.

Savor Your Food

Before you even take your first bite, consciously look over the plate and take it all in. Think about how those different flavors are going to entice your taste buds and about how the nutrients contained in the foods on your plate are going to make your body better. Take a moment to appreciate the effort that went into preparing the food and, if you are religious, thank the Creator for being the ultimate source of it.

Engage All of Your Senses

When that food heads your way, engage all of your senses in order to fully appreciate it. Take in the aroma, colors and texture. And then, when you put it in your mouth, see if you can identify all of the ingredients, including the sauces and seasonings.

Chew Your Food Thoroughly

Chewing your food well will help you to slow down in your eating. It will also maximize the release of digestive enzymes in the mouth. In addition, the more thoroughly you chew your food the less work your digestive system will have to do. And, according to recent research, the more you chew, the more satisfied you will be with your meal and the fewer overall calories you will consume.

Researchers have made links between chewing and enhanced cognitive benefits. Neural circuits in the brain connect the act of chewing with the hippocampus, which controls cognitive functioning. Chewing has also been shown to have a positive correlation with attention and focus.

Chew each bite a minimum of 10 times before swallowing it down.

SLOWING DOWN: THE ESSENCE OF MINDFUL EATING

A habit that many people have developed over their life's course is to shovel food into their mouth, one spoonful after the other, without a break. It's as if they're in a race to see who can finish eating first. Generally, these people tend to have too much fat on their bodies, whereas skinnier people will tend to eat more slowly. Let's find out why.

You get fuller faster when you eat slower. This is because your brain gets a chance to say "I'm full" at a faster rate, as opposed to just shoveling the food in and ending up with a stomach ache. For us to feel full, the brain needs to receive signals from hormones located in the gastrointestinal tract. This hormonal signaling system is a complex process by which leptin and chole-cystokinin (CCK) amplify the feeling of fullness. It takes a full twenty minutes, however, for the brain to get the signal that you are full. Shoveling the calories into your mouth at a rate of knots is going to massively over-supply your food needs. You will end up wearing the excess around your waist.

When we eat properly – i.e., slowly – the hormone leptin interacts with the neurotransmitter dopamine to produce a sensation of pleasure. When we eat too fast, however, dopamine is not released. We derive neither a feeling of fullness nor pleasure. This leads us to keep on eating.

Your stomach does not have teeth. So, everything that you put into it has to be broken down. When you eat fast, your body doesn't have a chance to process the food. As you chew it in your mouth, saliva begins the digestive process. By the time it goes down your throat, a large part of the digestive process has already been accomplished. But, when you simply swallow it down without chewing, you are placing undue stress on your gut. As a result, large pieces of unprocessed food can become trapped in the stomach, leading to gastric discomfort.

Eating too quickly can also lead to bloating. This problem occurs when too much air enters the digestive tract, as often happens when you eat too fast.

People who eat too fast tend not to enjoy their food as much. Food is one of the great pleasures in life. It deserves to be treated with respect, to be savored, relished and lingered over. Those who eat to complete are missing out on so much. They are depriving them-selves of the exquisite joy of flavor.

In addition to the pleasure of enjoying your food, slowing down your eating allows you to enjoy one of the other great joys of eating – socialization. Sharing a meal is perhaps the most universally accepted and widely enjoyed means of sharing time with others. In this regard, we can take a lesson from the Mediterranean world.

For centuries, the inhabitants of the 16 countries surrounding the Mediterranean have been experiencing a unique level of health, longevity and weight control. More and more people around the world have been joining them, not just to achieve optimum health but to shed excess body fat. The biggest difference between the way they eat and the way the Western world eats is that they take more time to enjoy and savor their meals.

ACTION PLAN

Eating slowly will take effort. In fact, it will require what has come to be known as mindful eating on your part. Mindful eating simply involves being consciously in the moment when you are eating. Here are four practical steps to help you to develop mindful eating and thus slow down and enjoy your food.

Step One

Plan to spend 30 minutes eating your larger meals. Get out of the mindset of dinner being an inconvenience that you have to get out of the way in order to get back to the TV set. Try to have the whole family sitting at the dinner table, turn off the TV (and your phone), and initiate a discussion. If your family isn't used to this, it may seem a little strange at first. You can help by having a strategy – ask each family member for their highlight (or lowlight) of the day.

Step Two

Count to ten before each bite. This will allow you to assess just how hungry you actually are. Think about it. If you're already feeling full, you are allowed to stop. Counting to ten will also provide time for you to fully digest the mouthful that has come before.

Step Three

Talk during your meal – when you're at a social gathering, don't think so much about the food. Think more about the company that you are with. You are eating so you can stay alive – and enjoy the association of your loved ones. Focusing on eating rather than communicating is akin to not seeing the forest for the trees!

Step Four

The body triggers its sensation for food and water based on diminished energy levels. These two sensations reach the brain together – and most people interpret them to be a sensation just to eat. The body does not send a separate signal for thirst and another one for food. As a result, we often reach for food when we should be reaching for water.

If we could separate these two sensations, then we would be at an immediate advantage in the battle to control our body fat levels.

Well, we can – and here's how:

Drink a glass of water before you eat.

When you do that, you will satisfy the body's need for hydration and you will prevent yourself from overeating. You should also drink water with your meal.

IDENTIFYING YOUR EATING HABITS

It's time now to take a close look at the eating habits that have developed in your life and that unconsciously dictate the way that you fuel your body. Not all of your eating habits will be detrimental. Some of them will be positive and you will definitely want to retain them. Others, however, will be clearly bad for you and you will be far better off without them. The first step to ditching them is identifying what they are.

7-Day Food Diary

In order to bring your unconscious eating habits to the forefront of your mind, you will have to do a little detective work. It begins with a food diary. Over the next 7 days, I want you to keep a diary of everything you eat.

You can either use a notebook as your food diary or download a food journal app. Here are the things you should make a record of:

- Date
- Time
- Place (e.g. at home in front of TV)
- Food item and quantity
- How you felt before and after eating
- Your hunger level before and after

6 Food Diary Tips

Record Everything

If it travels between your lips, it needs to be recorded in your food diary. That includes everything you drink as well as what you eat. Don't dismiss those nibbly snacks you eat on the run or even the sneaky mouthfuls you gulp down when cooking - record it all!

Break food meals down into ingredients. So, rather than writing' chicken sandwich', take note of how many pieces of bread you had, how much chicken and what, if any, sauces or other condiments you included.

Record your water intake as well.

Record Accurate Quantities

You should measure out the quantities of foods that you're eating with a pair of kitchen scales, along with measuring cups and bowls. The more accurate you are in recording your food intake, the easier it will be to analyze your habits once you're done.

Accurate Time and Place

Be as specific as you can in recording the time that you eat. So, rather than writing down 'afternoon snack,' jot down the actual time. This will help you to more accurately identify your eating patterns.

You also need to record where you eat in the home. Was it in front of the TV or at the dinner table, in bed, or at the kitchen aisle?

Emotional State

Were you feeling stressed immediately before eating? Was food your comfort? After the meal, did you actually feel comfort, or was guilt the overriding emotion? Whatever it was, write it all down.

Physical Reactions

Did you experience gas or bloating after the meal? Be sure to record all of your physical reactions to the food you eat.

Use the Hunger Gauge to Record your Hunger Level

The Hunger Gauge was created by nutritionists to help their clients train themselves to eat as a response to feeling hungry rather than as a result of social or other cues.

The hunger gauge has the following 6 levels to follow:

1. You are desperately hungry and experiencing clear physical signs of hunger, such as feeling shaky or faint.
2. You are very hungry; your stomach is rumbling and you feel a little tired.
3. You are moderately hungry; you have an appetite for food and a pleasant sense of anticipation.
4. You feel satisfied. You could perhaps be tempted to eat dessert, but it is not essential.
5. You are too full; you left it a little late to stop

eating because you couldn't resist the
temptation of another small helping.

6. You are very full; you ignored all the signs to
   stop eating and now feel weighed down. You
   may also experience indigestion and heartburn.

Note down a before and after Hunger Gauge rating for
every meal that you record in your food diary.

Listing Your Eating Habits

Once you have completed 7 days of your food diary,
you will have a key resource to help you identify your
eating habits. Take a piece of paper (or create a docu-
ment on your device) and divide it into two columns.
On the left-hand side, you will list all of the bad eating
habits that are part of your life. On the right-hand side,
note down all of the good nutrition habits that you
have developed.

Here is an example of the common good and bad habits that ingrain themselves as the rules of eating for many people . . .

Bad Eating Habits	Good Eating Habits
o Eating in front of TV o Eating too fast o Eating for comfort o Eating ready meals o Eating out too often o Hangovers and eating junk food o Fasting then binge eating o Weighing yourself too much o Going shopping hungry o Going back for seconds o Serving food at the table which makes getting seconds easier o Rewarding your good eating with desert too often o Snacking while cooking o Taking too long between meals o Portion sizes o Fixating on the bathroom scales o Takeaways o Weeks off, weekends on o The ' I've been good" rule	o Snacking on fruit o Eating frequent small meals o Eating slowly o Limiting red meat o Drinking water with meals

ANALYZE YOUR EATING TRIGGERS

Breaking the link between your emotional state and your food intake can be the first step to successful weight control. Recognizing that there is an emotional dimension to your eating will help you adopt healthy eating habits.

Having completed your food diary and listed your habits, you are in a great position to analyze both to identify your emotional eating triggers. Use your food diary to answer the following questions:

	YES	NO
Do you eat more when you are alone, such as when watching TV?		
Do you give yourself 'rewards' of chocolate or sweets if you have had a difficult day?		
If you have broken your diet and eaten a rich dessert, do you feel so upset that you might as well give up and eat what you like for the rest of the day?		
Does looking in the mirror or weighing yourself make you so depressed that you need a treat to cheer yourself up?		
Do you eat high fat energy foods, such as chips and chocolate to give you a pick-me-up boost when you are down?		

The Most Common Emotional Eating Triggers

Analyze your food diary in relation to these 6 most common emotional eating triggers:

Stress

When we get stressed, the body overproduces the hormone cortisol. Cortisol triggers a desire for salty, sweet and fried foods that deliver a quick energy boost. When under stress, we use food as a numbing strategy to distract us from the problem weighing on our minds. Research also shows that eating sugary foods can actually stimulate the pleasure centers in the brain in a similar way to such drugs like cocaine or heroin. Dopamine, the feel-good hormone, surges into the brain's pleasure center at the same time that endogenous opioids, the brain's natural painkillers, induce more positive feelings.

To identify if you are a stress eater, go back to your food diary and take a look at your Hunger Gauge numbers and your emotional state when eating various meals. If you can pinpoint several times during the week when you reached for sugar-laden foods at times when your hunger gauge was low and your emotional state was heightened, then you are a stress eater.

Burying Your Emotions

Can you identify periods during the week when you ate in order to bury disturbing emotions or memories? That piece of cake and cup of coffee becomes a soothing mechanism that allows us to put a band-aid over the troubling emotions that are gnawing away deep inside. You are, in effect, self-medicating with food. Meanwhile, the root emotional problem is festering - and you're gaining weight!

Boredom

Were there times during the week that you were doing something that you just couldn't get your mind excited about and then, as if on autopilot, you found yourself wandering to the fridge and opening the door in search of a snack? This is boredom eating. Boredom generates feelings of negativity, lack of fulfillment and frustration. Our natural reaction to those feelings is to find ways to reverse them. Food can easily become the trigger to doing so.

The thought of satisfying our taste buds with a delicious treat can be the counter to the negativity that boredom produces. Of course, that awesome taste is only momentary, so we eat more and more to keep feeling those positive emotions. But then what happens? Usually, we are plagued by feelings of disgust or guilt at our lack of self-control. And the boredom remains!

Social Influences

Food is the lubrication of social interaction. When we have visitors, or when we are visiting others, we often feel a social obligation to serve or bring an item of food. We eat it because it is served to us, not because we are hungry. Many people also eat out of nervousness when they are with others. Look back through your food diary to see if you can identify situations where you ate in social situations when your Hunger Gauge was higher than 3.

Binge Eating Disorder

Binge eating disorder, although not as prominently discussed as bulimia and anorexia nervosa, is actually the most common eating disorder in both the United States and the United Kingdom. In fact, binge eating disorder is three times more common in the United States than anorexia and bulimia combined.

Binge eating disorder is recognized by the Diagnostic and Statistical Manual of Mental Disorders (DSM-V), a standard classification used by health professionals, as a mental disorder. According to the DSM-V, binge eating disorder has the following characteristics:

- Recurring episodes of eating large amounts of food rapidly to the point of discomfort.
- During the eating, the person feels a sense of loss of control, as if they can't stop until there is no food left.
- Eating an amount of food that is significantly more than most would eat in similar circumstances in a short amount of time.
- Loss of control over how much/what one is eating, feeling like one cannot stop eating.
- Episodes of binge eating also must include at least three of the following characteristics: Eating rapidly and to the point of discomfort. Eating when one is not physically hungry. Eating alone so others do not know how much one is eating.
- Episodes followed by feelings of shame, guilt, disgust Distress around the binge-eating behavior.

Unlike other eating disorders such as bulimia nervosa, there are no compensatory activities involved, such as purging, taking laxatives, or excessive amounts of exercise. Binge eating has been described as a tornado that sweeps in and overtakes a person. When the urge to binge strikes, they feel unable to do anything about it. In a sense, the person is a bystander in their own body; all they can do is to watch themselves, as if from a distance, as they perpetuate the same desperate behavior time and again.

Binge eating is distinct from occasional overeating. It is accompanied by a complete loss of physical self-control where the person cannot possibly stop eating despite the physical discomfort that they feel.

There is no one identifiable cause of binge eating disorder. It results from a perfect storm aligning a number of contributing factors. These are a combination of genetic and environmental factors. With regard to the interplay between genetics and environment, Dr. Francis Collins of the US National Institute of Health commented, "genetics loads the gun; environment pulls the trigger."

The following factors work together to contribute to the development of the disorder:

- Genetic factors - recent research has

pinpointed a gene that may be a genetic risk factor for binge eating. This gene is called cytoplasmic FMR1-interacting protein 2 (CY-FIP2).

- Hormonal irregularities - sufferers of binge eating disorders have been shown to have increased levels of the hunger-inducing hormone ghrelin.
- Receiving the message from parents and others that food is a comfort and soothing mechanism.
- Being raised in an environment where there is a constant focus on dieting and weight loss.
- Life stressors that arise during teen years such as leaving home, relationship problems, academic pressures and other unfamiliar, challenging situations.
- Life transitions such as relationship breakup, moving to a new city or losing one's job.
- Depression or anxiety.
- Perfectionist tendencies.
- Addictive personality traits.

BREAKING FREE FROM BINGE EATING

Millions of people have managed to break the shackles of binge eating and so can you. Here are seven proven strategies that you can employ to overcome this condition:

Journaling

Journaling can be used as a therapeutic tool to help you when you get the urge to binge eat. Even though it will be difficult, rather than going with the surge of desire to begin eating, stop, breathe, count to 10 and reach for your journal. Now explore on paper the emotions that are driving your binge desire. Is it boredom? Loneliness? A painful memory or experience? Will food really be the panacea to this problem that your emotional driver is telling you that it will be?

When you write openly and honestly about your emotions, you will be forcing yourself to confront your emotions rather than running away from them.

Alternative Activities

By having an alternative coping mechanism in place prior to the binge urge overtaking you, you will be far more likely to resist it and not give in to the temptation. Your alternative activity could be to go for a walk, contact a support person, listen to your favorite music, exercise, take a bubble bath or practice a mindful breathing exercise.

Don't Skip Meals

It has been shown that planning out regular meal times and sticking to them is one of the proven ways to lessen the occurrence of binge eating. Plan your meals every three hours apart and stick to that schedule.

Practice Mindfulness

A meta-study that analyzed 14 studies found that the regular practice of mindfulness significantly decreased the incidence of binge eating. We have already discussed how mindful eating practices can help you to break free from bad eating habits. When it comes to binge eating, the key skill to develop is an awareness of your actual physical hunger level. Go back to the Hunger Gauge and rate yourself. If your rating is 4 or higher, forbid yourself from eating!

Drink Plenty of Water

Staying well hydrated will keep you feeling full throughout the day which will, in turn, make you less inclined to develop the binge eating urge. Drinking water before a meal will also make you less likely to binge. In one study, it was shown that consuming 500 mls of water before one meal per day decreased total daily caloric consumption by 13 percent in comparison to a control group.

Increase Fiber Consumption

Fiber is a great way to keep yourself full. That is because it adds bulk to your diet without adding extra calories. Not only will it help you to feel full sooner, but because it takes longer than other foods to move through your system, it will keep you full longer.

When fiber fills up your stomach, it stimulates receptors that send messages to your brain that tell you to stop eating.

Soluble fiber decreases enterohepatic recycling of bile acids which can decrease serum cholesterol levels. Insoluble fiber will add bulk to stools while also decreasing colon cancer risk.

An added benefit of soluble fiber is that, when it absorbs water, it forms a gel in the lower intestine. This slows the absorption of blood sugar. This, in turn, leads to lower insulin levels, which makes you less likely to store body fat.

Here's how you will benefit from these adaptations:

- Increased satiety
- Lowered blood fat and cholesterol
- Reduced risk of colon cancer
- Proper intestinal motility
- Enhanced gut health

When it comes to fruits and vegetables, the majority of the fiber is found in the skin, membrane and seeds. That's why you need to be eating fruits with the skin on.

If you are a woman, aim for 35 grams per day.
If you are a man, aim for 48 grams per day.

Be sure to drink plenty of water when you eat fiber. You'll need a minimum of eight glasses each day in order to keep the fiber moving through your system. Water, of course, also helps to keep you full.

Increase Protein Intake

Increasing your protein intake will help to fill you up and keep you satisfied throughout the day. The word protein is derived from the Greek *proteios*, meaning 'most important.' Along with carbohydrates and fats, it is one of the three macronutrients. We all know that protein is the key macro or muscle gain. Fewer people realize that it is also the main nutrient for satiety. Therefore, keeping a high protein intake will allow you to feel full all day long, which will make you far less likely to binge eat.

There are three ways that protein helps in this regard:

- It helps us to build lean muscle tissue. Once you

take away the water, muscle tissue is almost exclusively made of protein.

- Protein has a higher thermic effect than either carbohydrates or fat. During the process of digestion, some 25% of protein calories are used during digestion, compared to just 6-8% for carbs and 2-3% for fat.
- Protein fills you up, which helps you to go longer between meals without feeling hungry again.

There are a large number of studies that have shown that the combination of these three factors are effective factors in fat loss. People who are assigned to eat more protein lose more fat. Retain more muscle tissue, have less hunger and eat less total food.

In contrast, studies have shown that lower protein intake leads to overeating, fat gain, and muscle loss. Such results have led some researchers to propound the protein leverage hypothesis, which states that humans have the ability to keep track of how much protein we've eaten. This tracking system, it is claimed, is the ultimate controller of appetite. We eat more food when we have less protein in our meals and less when we have more.

According to the protein leverage hypothesis, then, hunger is really a quest for protein.

This protein leverage hypothesis seems to gel with what we see in society. Researchers have been scratching their heads for decades at the statistics which show that the wealthiest people in society are also the leanest, while the poorest people are the fattest. Of the three macronutrients, protein is the most expensive. So, if all that you eat is low-quality, mass-produced food, you'll need a lot more of it to reach your body's internal protein target.

Let's take a look at some of the exciting research that has ramped up protein's fat loss profile in recent years.

- *A 2014 study investigated the effects of protein intake on between-meal snacking and resultant weight loss. A group was given dairy protein every four hours as compared to a control group who only ate protein once per day but were also fed every four hours. Not only did the protein group resist the urge to graze between meals, their average weight loss after 28 days was 17% greater than the control group.*
- *A 2011 study of overweight and obese men by Leidy, et al. revealed that upping your protein intake while reducing carbs at every meal of the day resulted in a*

greater loss of body fat than only eating protein in the evening.

- *In 2011 a study was undertaken that showed that eating an ample amount of protein for breakfast significantly reduced food cravings throughout the remainder of the day. The test subjects were teenagers who normally skipped breakfast. They were exposed to visual food responses after being given a normal versus a high-protein breakfast. Those who were given the high-protein breakfast exhibited significantly greater neural resistance to the temptations shown to them.*

- *Many studies have shown that eating protein throughout the day preserves lean muscle mass when a person is losing body fat. This was seen in a 2008 study by Bopp, et al. which was published in the "Journal of the American Dietetic Association"*

- *A 2002 study specifically showed that eating more protein leads to an increase in fat loss.*

Another major advantage of protein?

Unlike carbohydrates or fats, taking in high levels of protein does not play havoc with your insulin levels!

BREAKING FREE FROM THE BINGE-RESTRICT CYCLE

The binge-restrict cycle is similar to the diet-relapse cycle that we discussed in the previous chapter, just on a more condensed time scale. Here's how it goes . . .

- You binge eat
- You experience feelings of guilt and shame
- You resolve to do better in the future
- You overcompensate by with some form of eating restriction
- You binge eat again

In order to break free from this cycle, you need to focus on the two key factors of physical hunger and negative emotions. After a binge eating episode, you need to resist the temptation to cut back on your next meal. Those feelings of guilt are only natural but realize that you do not have to be stuck into a cycle that perpetuates the problem. Focus on the next meal, which should be around 3 hours after your binge eating episode. This meal will probably be significantly smaller than usual, but it is vital that you have some food, just as you normally would.

You also need to break free from the categorization of food as good or bad. Food is just food. It should not have a moral tag attached to it. When you are able to de-stigmatize certain foods, you no longer view them as temptation foods. Often people binge on these so-called forbidden foods, but when you include them in moderation as part of a blanched eating plan, you take their power to tempt you into an overeating episode.

Another key to breaking out of the binge-restrict cycle is to not be too harsh on yourself. When you begin to experience those feelings of shame, put on the mental brakes. Remind yourself that you are not a robot. You are going to have slip ups, but you are smarter than falling back into the usual cycle.

Getting out of the binge-restrict cycle isn't easy. You probably won't succeed on the first occasion. Achieving long-term success is all about forgiving yourself when you slip up and being patient with yourself.

SUMMARY

In this chapter, you have closely analyzed the way you eat to identify your good and bad habits. You have kept a detailed 7-day food diary and then poured over it in order to bring to the forefront of your mind the unconscious habits that have built up over your lifetime to produce your personal rules of eating. We have also examined some of the more frequent habits that people create for themselves, both consciously and unconsciously.

We've discovered in this chapter that a powerful impetus to breaking free from the eating rules that enslave us is the concept of mindfulness. Mindful eating involves:

- Controlling what comes into the house
- Not allowing yourself to get too hungry
- Buying smaller plates
- Savoring your food
- Engaging all your senses
- Chewing your food thoroughly
- Slowing down

In the next chapter, we'll set about creating the new rules which will allow you to break free from your bad habits by adopting a refreshing new mindset.

6

BREAKING THE RULES

"Don't fear failure. In great attempts it is glorious even to fail"

— BRUCE LEE

Breaking free of the habits that have dictated the way you eat takes real effort. After all, you've been eating around a thousand meals a year for every year that you've been alive, so those habits are pretty well ingrained. The key to lasting change lies in undergoing a mental makeover. Unless you are able to achieve a complete mindset shift regarding food and your relationship with it, all of your actions will end up in frustration.

In this chapter, I'll provide you with a plethora of strategies, techniques and tips to allow you to develop the mindset to conquer your bad eating habits and create new rules that are guilt-free, making it far easier to maintain a healthy lifestyle.

ISSUES OF SELF ESTEEM

Research indicates that many people's bad eating habits are rooted in issues of poor self-esteem. With society's obsession with looks, that's hardly surprising. By the time the average young woman graduates from High School, she will have watched over 22,000 hours of television. That's nearly 2 and a half years of sitting in front of the TV 24 / 7. And during that time, she will have been deluged with images of sexy women with perfect bodies.

For many young women, this constant exposure to the perceived body ideal leads to a deeply seated subconscious connection between attaining a Sports illustrated Swimsuit body and love, happiness and fulfillment. And all of this has led to a distorted view of body image among many women. In a recent survey, 41% of female respondents described themselves as too fat, and 29% said that they were currently dieting. In fact, only 17% of them were overweight, according to body fat caliper testing.

The result of all of this media-fed body image control is that women have morphed their view of how they think they look onto their total self-image. A less than ideal self-body image, then, can result in some pretty toxic ideas about one's personal worth. Unless you consider yourself physically acceptable, you're likely to feel powerless, unworthy and unloved. That's pretty harsh when the view of what is acceptable is, in itself, an artificially constructed illusion. After all, the images we see in the magazines are airbrushed and photo-shopped to create an illusion of bodily perfection that simply does not exist. That's why most of us are looking at our body images through a distorted mirror. The following steps will help you to correct your view:

1. Start retraining yourself to forget about the false images that society has embedded in your brain about the body ideal. It has been designed for one thing only - to take your money. Your body is unique to you - focus on improving it bit by bit and forget everything else - and stop comparing yourself to others.
2. Judge your body by what it does for you rather than what you think it looks like. Your body is

an amazing living machine that deserves your respect. Cherish it, feed it so that it can do its best and NEVER put anything into it that will cause it damage.

3. Dig to uncover the real reasons behind any ongoing body image hang-ups that you have. What is it that is really holding you back from feeling good about yourself? Could it be that you were never praised as a child? Do you expect perfection from yourself? Whatever the issue is, make up your mind here and now to confront it rationally in the cold light of day. Acknowledge it. Accept it. Then remedy it.

4. Adopt a positive power base. You are about to engage upon an awesome weight management program that will allow you to finally achieve your physical goals. The mindset that you take into this endeavor is critical. Rather than coming from an "I'm broken and I need to be fixed" perspective, you should adopt the view that "I'm awesome and I deserve to be the best me that I can be."

5. Learn to judge yourself by what is really important. At the end of the day, your character is more important than your thigh size. Develop the qualities of love, compassion, empathy and hospitality and judge yourself

against these criteria. So make a list of positive non-body traits that you appreciate about yourself. Keep this close by and refer to it every day.

6. Realize that you are not alone. Everybody has doubts about how they look - including those supermodels who you've probably been judging yourself against for so long. Without their million-dollar make-up and airbrushed photoshoots, they're just like you.

7. View yourself as a whole person - you're more than just a sagging butt or beer belly. Look at yourself naked in the mirror and focus on the bits that you do like.

8. Surround yourself with positive people who clearly love themselves and will encourage you in the same regard. These people should love you for who you are, not what you have or how you look.

9. Be stronger than your negative thoughts. Shut them down, boot them out and clear the space for positivity. Any time you see a negative thought taking root, squash it and put a positive affirmation in its place.

10. Treat your body. Take a soothing bubble bath. Have a relaxing nap. Just find some time to chill out. Give back to the body that, up until now,

you've probably been berating and taking for granted.

UNDERSTANDING HUNGER

In order to break the bad eating habits that have accumulated over your life, you need to really understand what hunger is, what contributes to true hunger and how to differentiate between physical and emotional hunger.

When your stomach is empty of food, you experience hunger pangs in the form of contractions of the stomach wall. However, these stomach contractions are not only caused by lack of food. They may also occur as the result of your body's rhythms. The human body thrives on regularity and over the years, each of us has trained our body to eat at certain times. When we miss one of those feeding times, the body may react to physical cues like stomach contractions even though we are not busy.

The body's intake of food is regulated by two key hormones:

- Leptin
- Ghrelin

Leptin: The Hunger Controller

Leptin is one of the body's master hormones. Among its many other roles, leptin has the job of controlling how hungry you feel. This hormone is released by your fat cells and keeps a constant tally on your stored fat content and the amount of food you need to consume to provide the energy you need to function.

The higher the levels of leptin circulating through your system, the lower the levels of a hunger signaling hormone called NPY. A rodent study conducted by the Rockefeller Institute found that obese mice who were injected with leptin had a significantly reduced food intake and a boosted fat burn.

Research like this has led scientists to proclaim leptin as the 'gate-keeper of fat metabolism and the regulator of hunger'. As well as negating the hunger-boosting effects of NPY, it has also been shown to counter the hunger-stimulating effects of another hormone called anandamide. In addition, leptin is believed to stimulate the body's production of a hormone called a-MSH, which acts as an appetite suppressant.

When your body produces a normal level of leptin, the brain will receive appropriate messages to stop eating when you are full and you will be able to control your appetite. Because leptin is produced in our fat cells, the more stored body fat we have, the more leptin we will produce. You'd think that this will help overweight people to eat less. However, there's a problem.

When your body is overwhelmed by leptin production due to too many stored fat cells, you can develop what is known as leptin resistance. This is when the brain fails to respond to the signals it is receiving to stop eating. It has been overwhelmed by the hormone and metaphorically throws up its hands in despair. As a result, the body reverts to its starvation response of eating more and exercising less to preserve energy.

The following factors contribute to leptin resistance:

- eating too many simple carbohydrates
- high-stress levels
- high fructose
- overconsumption of grain
- lack of sleep

To avoid leptin resistance, be sure to follow these guidelines:

- Establish a sleep routine
- Get up at the same time each day
- Limit daytime napping:
- Get a handle on stress

- Cut down the coffee and alcohol
- Keep all technology out of your bedroom, including your smartphone
- Reduce your intake of sugar and processed carbohydrates
- Eat a protein with every meal
- Eat more healthy fats such as coconut oil, avocado and fish oil
- Eat your dinner 2-3 hours before bed time
- Perform high-intensity interval training (HIIT) workout 2-3 times per week

Ghrelin: The Hunger Initiator

Ghrelin is the yin to leptin's yang; it signals hunger while leptin signals fullness. Ghrelin is produced in an upper part of the stomach called the fundus. Its production increases when we are genuinely hungry. But hunger is not the only thing that leads to increased ghrelin secretion. So does lack of sleep. Research has even shown that simply looking at images of temping foods leads to enhanced ghrelin production.

Here are 3 ways to reduce ghrelin levels:

- Increase your intake of high fiber foods
- Eat lean protein at every meal
- Get 7-8 hours of sleep each night

THE TEN TYPES OF HUNGER

According to dietitians, there are 10 different types of hunger, each of which has a specific way to keep it in check. Let's consider each one briefly:

Eye Hunger

There's a reason why the most popular item pictured on Instagram is food; we eat with our eyes! When we see a beautifully presented food item, we feel an overwhelming urge to eat it immediately. I bet even looking at the front cover of this book made you want to go out and buy a candy bar!

The Solution: Stop looking - immediately divert your focus to a non-food item that brings you pleasure.

Ear Hunger

Hearing food, or simply hearing about it, can set our mouth to watering and make us feel that we simply must have that food now. It could be something as innocent as a person opening a packet of potato chips on the train or a delivery guy announcing Pizza's arrival next door.

The Solution: Again, the solution is to discipline

your mind to divert your attention to something else that will consume you and make you forget that false hunger cue.

Nose Hunger

Food sellers have been using the enticing smell of food for hundreds of years. Whether it's freshly baked banana bread, an oven-baked lasagna or freshly brewed coffee, that irresistible odor seems to entrance us, destroying our willpower and causing us to succumb to those temptations.

> The Solution: Make the effort to individually smell all of the foods on your plate. Take in the odor of each food as you consume it. When you do this, you will be teaching yourself to slow down, eat more mindfully and, as a result, you will eat less food overall.

Stomach Hunger

When your stomach is empty, it will 'growl' to let you know that it needs food. However, as previously mentioned, this stomach growling can also be due to the body's adherence to an established eating schedule rather than legitimate hunger.

The Solution: Use the Hunger Gauge that was introduced earlier to assess your actual as opposed to your perceived hunger level. Slow down in your eating and leave the table when you are not quite full.

Mouth Hunger

Mouth hunger is controlled by the taste buds. They create an intense desire for certain foods. These cravings are not a sign of actual hunger. However, they can be almost impossible to resist.

The Solution: Satisfy the craving with a small portion. When you do that, the craving will disappear. That is when you need to discipline yourself to stop.

Heart Hunger

Heart hunger can also be termed emotional hunger, where we eat for psychological rather than physical reasons.

The Solution: Practice the mindful eating strategies we have already considered. Reduce portion sizes and, once again, use the Hunger Gauge to assess your real state of hunger.

Cellular Hunger

Leptin and Ghrelin, introduced in the previous section, are the cellular controllers of appetite. The heavier a person is, however, the out of balance these hormones become in favor of Ghrelin, the hunger initiator.

> The Solution: Control your food regulating hormones by getting 7-8 hours sleep each night, eating lean protein at every meal and increasing fiber intake.

Stress Hunger

When we are stressed, we eat for comfort. Our minds are consumed without problems, so we don't have the energy to regulate what we are putting into our mouths. Rather, we eat for comfort.

> The Solution: Pause and force yourself to think of the consequences of your stress-induced food choices. Will they make you feel guilty later? Will you end up with a bloated stomach, gas and bloating? Is that what you really need?

Midnight Hunger

Many people wake during the night with a strong urge to go to the fridge and break open a tub of ice cream or pound back an extra-large piece of chocolate cake. This may be stress-related or a result of hormonal imbalance in favor of Ghrelin.

The Solution: Follow the sleep tips already given to increase the chances of not waking in the middle of the night. In case you do, have a small healthy snack on the bedside table, such as a handful of almonds or a banana.

Thirst Hunger

This last type of hunger should really be called mistaken hunger. We think we are hungry when we are, in fact, thirsty. The body triggers its sensation for food and water based on diminished energy levels. These two sensations reach the brain together – and most people interpret them to be a sensation just to eat. The body does not send a separate signal for thirst and another one for food. As a result, we often reach for food when we should be reaching for water.

The Solution: Drink a glass of water before you eat. When you do that, you will satisfy the body's need for hydration and you will prevent yourself from overeating.

3 STRATEGIES FOR ADOPTING HEALTHY EATING HABITS

From a psychological point of view, it is also more advantageous to add than to subtract. When it comes to your eating habits, thinking in terms of adding positive habits rather than getting rid of negative ones will put you at an advantage. Of course, in the process of adopting the good, you will be dropping the bad.

Here are three strategies that have been identified by psychologists when adopting healthy eating habits . . .

Manage Your Expectations

Many people set unrealistic expectations around their new eating goals. For one thing, they may expect to lose weight a lot faster than is realistic. The only thing that you should want to lose is stored body fat. A consistent weight loss of 1-2 pounds per week is realistic.

Aside from the drop in scale weight, people often have unrealistic emotional expectations. They may think that losing weight will bring them happiness. Yet, happiness is a multi-faceted diamond. Losing weight may contribute to that state but it will not assure it. However, if that is your expectation, there is a high chance that, when you don't find it, you will give up on your new eating habits and revert back to your old ways.

As a result, it is important to make your expectations about your new eating habits realistic.

Set Realistic Goals

Pressuring yourself with too many goals around your eating habits is a sure way to failure. The key to success is to slowly yet steadily implement one change at a time. Don't introduce a new habit until you have got on top of the previous one.

Focus on Adding, Not Removing, Foods

When you remove anything, you can't help but have a slight feeling of deprivation. Avoid this by concentrating on adding healthy foods to your day rather than excluding unhealthy foods. If you introduce the habit of having a mid-morning snack of sliced apple and walnuts, for example, you will, without focusing on it, have removed the habit of chowing down on cookies as your snack of choice.

Get Back on the Horse

Never forget that you are a human being, not a robot. Your progress toward healthy eating will not be linear. There will be setbacks and there will be times when you feel like a failure. Realizing and accepting that at the outset is critical to success.

When you slip up and revert to eating the way you know you shouldn't, you need to isolate that episode and move on from it. Don't beat yourself up over your slip-up. Simply accept it, get back on the horse and keep moving forward.

HOW HABITS WORK

Let's conclude this chapter with a consideration of how habits are formed. This will allow you to strategically use each of the habit formation stages as the basis for adding new habits and dismantling old ones. I'll then provide you with a dozen habits that you should begin to adopt at any age, but especially if you are over the age of 40.

There are three steps to the creation of habits:

1. The Trigger
2. The Behavior
3. The Reward

The Trigger

Everything starts with the habit trigger. You need to take the time to initiate the right triggers. There are four main types of triggers that cure our habits:

Location

Our environment has a powerful effect on our actions. By manipulating your environment in favor of a desirable outcome, you will be far more likely to follow through with the habit you are trying to introduce. For example, you will be more likely to introduce the habit of eating more fruit as a snack by purchasing beautiful fresh fruit every few days and displaying it on your kitchen counter than if you allow the bananas to go black and mushy and hardly ever top up your apple and citrus supply.

Time

Connect your new habit to a certain time of the day. You probably already have a set time to get up in the morning. Let's stay it is 6:30am. If you are trying to introduce the habit of drinking more water, tie the habit to the clock so that at 6:35am you drink a full glass of water. You might not feel like drinking water at that time but you will do it anyway because you know that is what your body needs and you are regulated by the clock.

Prior Actions

Connecting a habit to a prior action is known as habit stacking. It involves introducing a new habit by piggy-backing off another habit or routine that you have already ingrained in your life. For example, you may have the routine of walking to the bus each morning. If you are trying to develop the habit of eating more fruit, pair it with grabbing an apple on your way out the door.

The Actions of Others

Other people have a huge influence on our actions and our habits. As far as it depends upon you, surround yourself with people who are also trying to eat in a more healthy manner. Explain the reasons for your desire to break your bad eating habits to your loved ones and ask for their support. Even if they don't fully embrace your new ways of eating, knowing that they are behind and will not do things to jeopardize your goals makes a big difference.

The Behavior

The behavior or 'action' is simply the response to these triggers. As previously stated, if you use the correct triggers, you are likely to follow up with the intended behavior. For example, if you display fresh fruit in the kitchen, you are far more likely to eat it than if it is hidden away in the fridge. You are also using healthier foods like fresh fruit and nuts as a replacement to snacking on processed, high sugar treats. If you don't buy these unhealthy foods at the store, you are limiting your chances of eating them on a regular basis.

The Reward

The habit reward stage is built on the established principle of operant conditioning, which states that, if we receive a positive feeling after doing something, we will continue doing it. When it comes to adopting your nutritional habits, you will feel immediate psychological rewards in terms of feeling better about yourself and your ability to master nutritional temptation. Allow yourself to go there mentally, congratulating yourself for what you are achieving. You will also experience improved physical health almost immediately. You will feel less bloated, sluggish and weighted down. Problems you may have had with gas and acid reflux will begin to lessen and you will start to lose those extra pounds. Recognize and acknowledge these rewards for your actions.

Your brain will soon understand that if it sees the cue and does the action, it will get the reward. When you think about it, switching from a bad habit to a good habit doesn't have to require changing all three of these steps. If you stick with the same trigger and reward but simply switch out the action in the middle, you should, theoretically, be able to transform a bad habit into a good habit.

Let's consider an example to see how this might work in practice:

> *You're at work and it comes to your lunch break. Everyone else automatically heads outside for a cigarette break. But you are trying to break the smoking habit, you head out for a 10 minute walk in the fresh air.*

We see that the cue remains the same- the lunch bell. The activity changes. But the reward, getting out of the work environment and relaxing the mind remains the same. You also get the extra benefit of fresh air, which you can't exactly claim on a cigarette break!

CHANGING A BAD HABIT TO A GOOD HABIT

Let's stick with the bad habit of smoking to analyze the change process in a little more detail.

There are all sorts of cues for a person to light up a cigarette. These might include going outside, being stressed or just being bored. The first step to conquering your bad habit is to write down all of the cues that lead you to reach for a cigarette.

Next, you need to find a replacement habit that is somewhat similar but better for you. An example would be to pop a piece of gum into your mouth. This makes sense when it comes to defeating the smoking habit because research tells us that the smoking habit has a lot to do with the fixation on the mouth. You are breathing in and out and holding the cigarette between your lips. So, replacing it with an activity that is also mouth-centric, like chewing gum, makes sense.

The replacement activity needs to also provide a reward. This might require a bit of thinking. You need to be careful because people often replace one bad habit with another. A common one is to go from smoking to eating. This results in excess calorie consumption and weight gain.

One strategy that you could utilize is to put aside the money that you would have previously spent on cigarettes to provide a tangible reward. If you used to smoke a pack of cigarettes a day, at an average cost of $6.50 per pack, that's a little under $50 a week that you'll be able to put aside. Maybe you can take your partner out for a restaurant meal once a fortnight or go out for a movie. Even though the reward will not be immediate when you are replacing the habit, it will still be powerful to provide the positive reinforcement that you need to succeed.

A DOZEN NUTRITIONAL CHANGES TO EMBRACE BEFORE YOU TURN 40

When you move into your fourth decade, your body's nutritional needs change. That's because you are now dealing with the effects of age-related hormonal and physical changes that are occurring inside your body. The following 12 healthy changes to adopt in your 40s come directly from the top doctors, nutritionists and mental health professionals on the planet. Remember to add them one at a time and not to move on to the next one until the current habit is ingrained.

Change #1: Avoid blood sugar spikes by snacking on lean protein, nuts and fruit as an energy pick-me-up rather than processed high glycemic carb foods.

Change #2: Cut your caffeine consumption back to between 50-80 mg per day; that's the equivalent of one medium-sized cup of coffee. Replace your other previous coffee breaks with water.

Change #3: Start supplementing with fish oil and a daily multivitamin that contains at least 2.4 mcg of Vitamin B12.

Change #4: Cut out empty calories; your body can no longer get away with several portions of junk each week! After 40 you need to make smarter choices about how you fuel your body. Go for the most nutrient-dense foods that provide maximum value for the minimum caloric cost.

Change #5: Plan to eat 20-30 grams of protein per meal. That will fill you up and help offset age-related muscle wasting.

Change #6: Consciously think about getting more antioxidants in the form of vegetables, fruits, nuts and beans.

Change #7: Increase your intake of omega-3 fatty acids by including eggs, fatty fish, nuts and avocados in your diet.

Change #8: Set a priority on including high fiber foods in your diet. This will help with digestion and elimination as well as keeping you regular. Fiber also fills the stomach so that you are less likely to graze between meals.

Change #9: Look after your bone health by including 3 servings of dairy per day. This will provide you with about 1000 mg of calcium. If you are vegan or don't do well with dairy, get your calcium from sweet potatoes, baby carrots, green beans, broccoli and oranges.

Change #10: Reduce your plate size. Go down from 12 inches to 9 inch diameter plates and your daily caloric consumption will reduce by a quarter!

Change #11: Start a Food Journal. This is a great way to keep yourself accountable and to begin thinking mindfully about what you are eating and why. If you get into the habit of recording everything you've eaten in the early evening, you will also be far less likely to eat rubbish food before going to bed.

Change #12: Strength Training. Beginning a regular, balanced strength training program before the age of 40 will allow you to face the future head-on. Strength training has been shown to be effective at combating every single one of the biomarkers of aging. Research also shows that people who are regularly exercising are far more likely to be successful at making long-term positive changes to the way they eat.

SUMMARY

In this chapter, we have established the mental foundation to break bad eating habits and adopt new, healthier nutritional habits. We identified issues of self-esteem as being at the root of many people's poor eating habits and then provided 10 strategies to improve self-esteem and break away from society's body obsession.

We then took a deep dive into what true hunger is and how to differentiate between physical and emotional hunger. We identified the two key hormones that regulate hunger . . .

- Leptin
- Ghrelin

In order to balance these key hormones, you need to:

- Get 7-8 hours of sleep each night
- Eat protein with every meal
- Do High-Intensity Interval Training (HIIT) Workouts
- Eat more high-fiber foods

We then identified the 10 types of hunger as identified by dietitians along with strategies to control each of them. Next, we focused on strategies for adopting healthy eating habits, including managing expectations, setting realistic goals and focusing on adding rather than removing foods and getting back on track when you slip up.

The three parts of the Habit Loop were identified . . .

- The Trigger
- The Behaviour

- The Reward

… and I showed you how they can be used to change a bad habit into a good habit.

We concluded this chapter with a dozen nutritional changes that everyone by the age of 40 should embrace.

In the next chapter, we focus on the importance of food as energy, as well the vital role that hydration and recovery play in combating many of the factors that contribute to bad eating habits.

STEP THREE. PRACTICAL SOLUTIONS

7

FUEL, HYDRATION & RECOVERY

"Your body is your most priceless possession. Take care of it"

— JACK LALANE

W ithout energy, you will not survive. The one and only source of that life-giving fuel is food. That food comes into your body in the form of three macro, or large, nutrients:

- Carbohydrates
- Proteins
- Fats

As those fuel sources are digested in the body, they are broken down into glucose, amino acids and fatty acids. These compounds enter the bloodstream and are then utilized in the process of respiration, which creates adenosine triphosphate (ATP), the main fuel that our bodies use.

There are three ways that the body creates ATP. These three energy systems are:

- The ATP-PCR system
- The glycolytic system
- The oxidative system

The first two of these energy systems do not require oxygen, while the third one does. As a result, it is also known as the aerobic (literally 'living in air') system.

The ATP-PCR system allows for exercise between 5-15 seconds. The ATP stored in the muscle will power up to the first five seconds. The salt phosphate (PCR) attaches to ATP to provide another 10 seconds or so of energy.

Once the ATP-PCR system is used up, the body switches to the glycolytic system. Now the body relies upon glycogen, which is the broken-down form of carbohydrate, to make ATP. This is achieved through the process of glycolysis. During glycolysis, lactate is produced, along with hydrogen ions. These are responsible for the muscle burn and fatigue you feel when sprinting or lifting heavy weights.

The glycolytic system will sustain you for up to two minutes of exercise. After that, the body switches to the oxidative system. With this system, ATP is produced using two mechanisms:

- The Krebs cycle
- The electron transport chain

The oxidative system produces ATP more slowly than the other two systems, but it will provide energy for a greater duration. This explains why you can run slowly for a long period of time, but sprint for only a short period of time, before you are exhausted.

SPOTLIGHT ON THE MACRONUTRIENTS

The amount of energy stored in food is measured in calories. In terms of the macronutrients:

- Carbohydrates contain 4 calories per gram
- Proteins contain 4 calories per gram
- Fats contain 9 calories per gram

As a guide, the average adult male needs 2500 calories daily and, and the average woman needs 2000 calories daily to maintain a healthy weight. This amount will vary depending on how much you exercise (you will require fewer calories if you are sedentary than if you are very active).

Along with providing energy, all of these macronutrients have specific roles in your body that allow you to function properly.

Carbohydrates

Carbohydrates (or carbs) are the only one of the three macronutrients that are not essential for life. Though the glucose which it provides is essential, this can also be obtained from fats and proteins. Getting glucose from carbs, though, is faster and more efficient.

Carbohydrates can be classified as either simple or complex. Simple carbs are quickly absorbed into the body. They cause an immediate surge in blood glucose levels. This effect is pronounced when you eat carbs by themselves, which is one reason you should avoid doing this. The rate at which carbohydrates are absorbed and digested has a direct bearing on energy levels, body composition and overall health. Carbs that are 'time-released' from low glycemic index foods will keep you fuller for longer, balance out your blood sugar and provide a slow release of energy.

Carbohydrates with a low glycemic-index are found in vegetables, fruits, legumes, and whole grains and should predominate in the diet over simple carbs such as fruit, dairy products, and processed and refined sugars like candy, table sugar, syrups, and soft drinks.

Neither simple nor complex carbs are good or bad. However, your dietary focus should be on complex carbs, with simple carbs being reserved as sometimes or treat foods.

Complex carbs don't provide the immediate energy that you get with simple carbs. But nor do they cause havoc with your blood sugar levels. They are more substantial and filling than simple carbs and usually contain fiber, which is a form of carbohydrate that is indigestible to humans and is extremely important for our gut health.

Complex carbs can be further divided into starches and fibrous vegetables.

Plants store energy in the form of starch. The following are the most common starchy foods that you should include in your diet:

- Yams
- Whole Grains
- Bread

- Pulses
- Beans
- Corn
- Pumpkin
- Sweet Potatoes

Because the human body can digest all of the calorie energy in starchy carbs, they are said to be more calorie-dense than fibrous carbs.

It is vital, however, that a healthy nutrition plan includes a healthy supply of fibrous vegetables. Here are some common types of fibrous carbs that should also feature on your plate regularly:

- Broccoli
- Asparagus
- Cauliflower
- Spinach
- Lettuce
- Brussels sprouts
- Tomatoes
- Cucumber
- Peppers
- Onions
- Bok choy
- Kale
- Mushrooms

- Courgettes

Fats

Fats are organic molecules that are made of carbon and hydrogen. They join together in long chains called hydrocarbons. The way that these hydrocarbons form and their length determines the type of fat that is created.

The simplest unit of fat is the fatty acid. Depending on the number of hydrogens affixed to each carbon along the hydrocarbon chain, two different types of fatty acids are formed:

- Saturated
- Unsaturated

The difference between saturated and unsaturated fatty acids comes down to their bond structure. Saturated fatty acids do not contain any double bonds and they have a full complement of hydrogen molecules associated with each carbon molecule.

Unsaturated fatty acids do contain double bonds and have fewer hydrogen molecules. They are able to be broken down into monounsaturated fatty acids, in which only one carbon is unsaturated, and polyunsaturated fatty acids, in which more than one carbon is unsaturated.

Fatty acids can be joined together to form what is known as triglycerides. This occurs when three fatty acids join together with a glycerol molecule. Triglycerides are the main component of fat in the diet. They are also the major form of storage fat on the body.

Saturated fats are found mainly in animal-based foods, whereas unsaturated fats are predominant in plant-based foods.

Because many people eat a lot of animal-based foods and few plant-based foods, they have an imbalance in favor of saturated fats. This is often combined with a high carbohydrate intake, which appears to accentuate the ill effects of a high saturated fat intake. It is recommended that our unsaturated to saturated fat intake ratio should be around 65:35.

Common sources of saturated fats include:

- Meat
- Poultry
- Butter
- Cheese
- Palm Oils

When we consume fats, the process of digestion involves the breaking down of triglycerides into fatty acids and glycerol. The fatty acids are an important source of energy for the body. In fact, a gram of fat has more than twice the energy potential of a gram of carbohydrate. Fats are also used for the manufacture and balance of hormones, the formation of cell membranes, and fat-soluble vitamins A, D, E and K.

Proteins

Every part of your body, from your big toe to the hairs on your head, is constructed from protein. Proteins are made up of chains of amino acids. The quality of a protein depends on its completeness according to its amino acid profile. There are 20 amino acids that are needed by the human body for growth. These 20 amino acids form into an untold number of configurations to make all manner of molecules. Eleven of the twenty can be manufactured within the human body.

That leaves nine amino acids that have to come from the foods we eat. These are the essential amino acids:

- Histidine
- Isoleucine
- Leucine
- Valine
- Lysine

- Methionine
- Phenylalanine
- Threonine
- Tryptophan

Animal protein sources, such as meat, fish, poultry, eggs, milk and cheese, are considered to be complete proteins. There are some plant protein sources that are also complete in their amino acid profile. These include:

- Quinoa
- Buckwheat
- Hempseed
- Amaranth

Most plant sources of protein, however, are considered to be incomplete because they do not contain all of the essential amino acids. In order to get all of the essential amino acids, people who follow a plant-based nutrition plan should use complementary protein choices. Combining wheat or rice, which are limited in lysine, with legumes, which are limited in tryptophan, can provide a full essential amino acid intake.

Water

Your body thrives on water. We use water in every cell, organ and tissue in order to maintain our body functions. In fact, according to the US Geological Survey, 60% of your body is water. To put that another way, if you're a 150-pound man, 90 of those pounds (40 liters) are water!

Water has many roles in the body, including:

- Regulating body temperature
- Lubricating joints
- Moistening tissues for mouth, eyes and nose
- Protecting body organs and tissues
- Preventing constipation
- Helping dissolve minerals and other nutrients to make them accessible to the body
- Reducing the burden on the kidneys and liver by flushing out waste products
- Carrying nutrients and oxygen to the cells

Without the right amount of water, your body simply will not function properly. However, we lose water just by going about our daily lives. If our 150 lb man does nothing all day except sit and breathe, he will still lose around 1.5 L of water over the course of the day through sweating, urination, and respiration. The more activity he does, the more water he will lose. If he does not replace this water, he will become dehydrated.

Dehydration reduces the amount of blood in the body, forcing the heart to pump harder in order to deliver oxygen-bearing cells into our muscles. For our 150 lb man, losing 3-5 L (just 1/8 of his body's water) of water will result in headaches and lethargy. After losing 6-7 L of water, mental impairments become apparent. If he loses much more than 10 L, he will go into shock and die. It is therefore vitally important that water lost is replenished.

So, how do you meet your daily hydration needs?

You have probably heard the often-cited recommendation to consume 8 glasses of water per day. That is a good guideline to aim for. The best way to meet that goal is to carry a water bottle with you and regularly sip from it, with the goal of getting through two and a half 750 ml (25 oz) bottles over the course of the day.

THE IMPORTANCE OF SLEEP

You enter your bedroom, change into your pajamas and slip between the sheets. You snuggle into the fetal position, each muscle in your body loosening and relaxing and your mind emptying. Your head sinks into the comfort of your pillow as you relish this time of recuperation – your daily reward for a hard day's work. You close your eyes and drift into a peaceful, regenerative sleep.

In those moments before you fall asleep, melatonin is produced in your brain. Its job is to slow down your metabolism. As melatonin begins coursing through your body, your body temperature drops slightly, blood flow to the brain is reduced and your muscles slowly start to loosen and become flaccid.

You now gently move into the first stage of what is known as non-REM or non-Dream sleep. This is shallow sleep during which your brain waves perform in rapid, irregular patterns. Your muscles become totally relaxed and your metabolism slows further as more melatonin is released. You will go through this first stage several times during the course of the evening. Each one will last between 30 seconds and seven minutes.

You now cruise straight into stage two, which has been called true sleep. About 20% of your night will be spent in this stage. It is characterized by enlarged brain waves as your mind produces fragmented ideas and visuals. Yet you are in a deep sleep and have no awareness of your surroundings.

Stages three and four are known as the delta zone. You are moving from deeper into deepest sleep. During this phase, the majority of the blood coursing around your body is being directed to your muscles. Your brain produces enlarged, slow waves. You are now in the power stage of sleep. Someone trying to wake you would have the most difficulty during stage four sleep. That's because it's during this phase that your body is replenishing, recovering and repairing itself. Ideally, you will spend about 50% of the night in stage four sleep.

About two hours into your slumber, your eyes will start to quiver rapidly backward and forwards. You are entering what scientists have dubbed Rapid Eye Movement (REM) sleep. Researchers have discovered that during a good night's sleep, you will move in and out of the REM stage several times. It is during REM sleep that you dream, as more blood is redirected to your brain. In fact, during REM your brain is acting almost as if you were awake.

Throughout the night, you are constantly moving through the 5 stages of sleep – the four non-REM stages and REM – such that every 90 minutes you are in REM sleep. Each time you enter REM, however, the phase lasts longer.

After seven to eight hours of uninterrupted sleep, you will go through six or seven complete sleep cycles. You will wake up refreshed, invigorated and ready to seize the coming day.

The Consequences of Broken Sleep

It should be clear from the above that several portions of broken sleep do not add up to the same amount of uninterrupted sleep. If you are waking up several times during the night, you may not be giving yourself enough time to reach stage four non-REM or REM sleep. Then, when – and if – you drift back to sleep again, you start back at Phase One again. That's why people who suffer from broken sleep can suffer from fatigue, apathy and depression the next day.

When you are regularly denied the cyclical 5 phases of sleep, you develop what is called **sleep debt.** Sleep debt prevents you from getting the amount of REM sleep that you need. REM sleep is vital for mental health. Bodily repair takes place during Stage 4 of non-REM sleep. Without these vital repair stages, you will suffer from:

- Reduced attention span
- Memory and vocabulary loss
- Diminished analytical thinking ability
- Diminished creativity

- A diminished sense of humor and social skills
- Reduced communication and decision skills
- Diminished resistance to viruses
- Reduced work productivity
- Enhanced risk-taking
- Increased likelihood of heart attack
- Increased susceptibility to diabetes
- Increased susceptibility to cold and flu
- Increased irritability
- Fat gain
- General lethargy
- Fatigue
- Lack of interest in what is going on around you

That is quite an ominous list. However, many people who are accustomed to getting by on a minimum amount of sleep are not even aware of many of these effects. Even though constant sleep shortage may diminish their mental faculties – specifically their alertness and reaction time – they operate under the mistaken impression that they haven't been affected at all. One result of this deceptive thinking can be seen in the carnage that occurs every day on our motorways.

Establishing Good Bedtime Habits

Clear Out Bedroom Junk

Your bedroom should be for two things only - sleep and sex. If you have TV in the bedroom, or you take your phone to bed with you, you will be tempted to use them, causing havoc to your sleep plans.

Establish a Wind-Down Routine

If you go to bed with your head buzzing and your stomach still trying to digest your last meal, you are going to struggle to get to sleep. A wind-down routine that begins a few hours ahead of hitting the sack can make all the difference.

Plan to finish your last meal three hours before going to bed. Then, about an hour and a half before going to bed, find something soothing to do in dim light. You could read a book, listen to music, work on a jigsaw puzzle, or anything else that you find calming and relaxing.

Follow your relaxing hour up with a warm bath. Stay in the water for at least ten minutes and get out at least an hour before bedtime. This will allow your core body temperature to cool down.

With half an hour to go before bedtime, fill out a 'To-Do' journal, in which you write down everything you need to do the next day. This will mean that you will spend less time agonizing about what you need to be doing the next day in the middle of the night.

Eating Your Way to a Good Night's Sleep

Changing what and when you eat can help you to get a better night's sleep. Here are the key facts you need to know:

- Do not eat within, ideally, three hours of bedtime.
- Cut back on sugar, sugary treats, drinks and desserts, particularly shop-bought ones.
- Get more fiber into your diet by switching to brown rice and by eating more quinoa, bulgar, whole rye, wholegrain barley, wild rice, buckwheat, lentils and beans.
- Full-fat yogurt is a good source of probiotics. Add blackberries, strawberries or blueberries for flavor and sprinkle in some walnuts.
- Eat such oily fish as salmon, tuna, and mackerel, which are rich in omega-3 fatty acids, two to three times per week.

SUMMARY

In this chapter, we have focused on the biological reason we eat, which is to provide the energy needed to power us through our lives. We've discovered that adenosine triphosphate (ATP) is the primary fuel that our bodies use. There are 3 ways that the body manufactures ATP:

- The ATP-PCR system
- The glycolytic system
- The oxidative system

We then shone a spotlight on the 3 key macronutrients. Carbohydrates, which provide glucose, are the most efficient energy source. Carbs also provide fiber, which promotes satiety and boosts gut health.

Fats can be either saturated or unsaturated. Fats, in the form of triglycerides, are the major form of fat storage in the body. Protein, in the form of amino acids, makes up the building material of the body. Humans cannot manufacture 9 of the 20 amino acids that are most crucial to the body. Foods that contain all 9 of the essential amino acids are known as complete proteins.

Finally, we touched on hydration and rest. Water is essential to the efficient functioning of the body – you should aim to drink 8 glasses of water each day. Sleep is also crucial to overall health, being especially important for renewing energy levels and relieving stress.

8

SO, WHAT SHOULD MY MEALS LOOK LIKE?

"Your diet is like a bank account. Good food choices are good investments"

— BETHENNY FRANKEL

W e now come to the part of this book where the rubber meets the road. Having gone in-depth on the bad eating habits that develop over our lives, and then provided the strategies to break free of those habits, we are able to zero in on the nutritional habits that will revolutionize the way you eat and transform your energy levels, your health and the way your body looks and feels.

Over the past half-century, various governmental agencies around the world have released a number of nutritional templates, each of which was lauded as the best way for everyone to eat. The USDA Food Pyramid was introduced in 1992 and eagerly adopted across the nation. Unfortunately, its advice was seriously flawed as the result of agricultural business lobbying.

This food pyramid was based on the premise that all carbohydrates are good for our health. That is why carb-based foods such as bread and pasta formed the wide base of the pyramid. At the other end of the pyramid, representing its narrow tip, were fats, which were to be consumed sparingly. However, it wasn't long before researchers began to identify issues with this advice. A variety of updates have been made in the official US Dietary Guidelines since then, and current guidance suggests following Harvard's Healthy Eating Plate. This is a colorful plate-shaped graphic created by Harvard Health Publishing, a division of Harvard Medical School, and is based on the most up-to-date nutritional research. It has the added benefit that it is not influenced by food industry or agriculture policy and is the way that I would recommend trying to eat on a daily basis.

The Healthy Eating Plate is divided into four unequal-sized sections:

- The largest section is **green** for vegetables
- Two-quarters of the plate are **orange** for protein and **brown** for whole grains
- The smallest section is **red** for fruits

In addition to the plate, there is a glass representing water, a bottle representing healthy plant oils, and a running figure representing exercise. The guidance suggests that you skip sugary drinks entirely, limit milk and dairy products to a maximum of two servings daily, and fruit juice to one small glass per day.

Let's take a closer look at the foods that make up each of these sections.

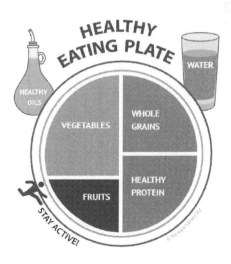

PLANT-BASED FOODS: VEGETABLES, WHOLE GRAINS & FRUITS

As the Healthy Eating Plate suggests, plants should form the basis of your diet. Both fruit and vegetables contain the vitamins, minerals, and other micronutrients that your body needs in order to run in tip-top condition! Plus, the trillions of microbes living in our gut (known as our gut microbiome, which is essential in helping to control digestion and boosting your immune system) require different types of plant foods to thrive. Increasing the diversity of the plant-based foods we eat helps to strengthen our gut microbiome, which in turn results in better health!

Furthermore, plant-based foods are naturally high in fiber. Though not officially classified as essential, fiber is an extremely important nutrient. There are two forms of fiber; soluble and insoluble.

Soluble fiber is found in such foods as oats and oat bran, dried beans and peas, nuts, barley, flax, fruits like oranges and apples, and carrots. Insoluble fiber is found in vegetables such as green beans and dark green leafy vegetables, fruit skins and root vegetable skins, whole-wheat products, seeds, and nuts. Both types of fiber, while indigestible, play important dietary roles:

- Fiber slows down the breakdown of carbohydrates into glucose. This helps to balance out blood sugar levels and prevent sharp spikes in insulin release.
- Fiber helps us feel fuller for longer by slowing down the release of hunger-promoting hormones.
- Soluble fiber helps to reduce unhealthy cholesterol levels.
- Insoluble fiber adds bulk to stools and decreases colonic transit time, which helps to boost our overall gut health.

Plus, an increase of just 8 g of fiber per day has been linked with:

- 19% reduction in risk of heart disease.
- 15% reduction in risk of type 2 diabetes.
- 8% lower risk of colon cancer.

Though the minimum recommended intake for fiber is 25 grams per day, the optimal amount seems to be closer to 35 grams per day for women and 48 grams per day for men.

However, just 10% of us are getting the recommended amount of fiber daily!

So, how do we ensure we get adequate plant diversity on our plate?

You may have heard of the World Health Organisation's recommendation of '5 A Day', as eating 400 g of fruit and vegetables (or five portions of fruit and veg) has been shown to lower the risk of serious health problems such as heart disease, stroke, and even some forms of cancer. In 2021 research conducted by at Harvard T. H. Chan School of Public Health found that eating two servings of fruit and three servings of vegetables is associated with lower mortality rates.

Furthermore, researchers at King's College London have also suggested that all fruits, veggies, wholegrains, legumes (beans and pulses), nuts and seeds, and herbs and spices count to this total!

Here are some tips to help you increase your plant-based foods intake:

- Always choose whole grains over refined grains, which have been stripped of valuable nutrients (including fiber) during processing. This could be as simple as switching from white to wholegrain bread, keeping the skin on your vegetables when cooking, or sprinkling seeds onto your salads.
- Place fruit where you can see it, e.g. in a bowl

on the kitchen counter, or chopped up (fruit salad style) in a bowl in the fridge.

- Go exploring down the produce aisle and regularly try new vegetables.
- Aim to eat the rainbow!

Add Color to Your Plate with the Food Rainbow

Filling your plate with a variety of colors does more than look good. Each of those colors represents a different nutrient profile that nourishes and enriches your body. Make it your aim to include two to three colors on your plate at each meal.

Here are the key foods to consume in each color range and the key nutrients they provide:

Red

- Tomatoes
- Pink Guava
- Grapefruit
- Red Bell Peppers

Key Nutrients: Lycopene, Folate, Potassium, Vitamin C, Vitamin B6

Orange and Yellow

- Carrots
- Sweet Potatoes
- Yellow Bell Peppers
- Bananas
- Pineapple
- Tangerines
- Pumpkin
- Winter Squash
- Corn

Key Nutrients: Carotenoids, Fiber, Folate, Potassium, Vitamin A, Vitamin C

Green

- Spinach
- Kale
- Broccoli
- Asparagus
- Avocados
- Green Cabbage
- Brussels Sprouts
- Green Herbs
- Green Bell Peppers

Key Nutrients: Chlorophyll, Carotenoids, Indoles, Fiber, Folate, Iron, Potassium, Vitamin A, Vitamin K1, Vitamin C, Vitamin B6

Blue & Purple

- Blueberries
- Blackberries
- Concord Grapes
- Red/Purple Cabbage
- Eggplant
- Plums
- Elderberries

Key Nutrients: Anthocyanins, Fiber, Manganese, Potassium, Vitamin B6, Vitamin C, Vitamin K1

Dark Red

- Beets
- Prickly Pears

Key Nutrients: Betalains, Fiber, Folate, Magnesium, Manganese, Potassium, Vitamin B6

White & Brown

- Cauliflower
- Garlic

- Onions
- Mushrooms
- Parsnips
- White Potatoes
- Apples
- Pears
- Chicory
- Cucumber

Key Nutrients: Anthoxanthins, Fiber, Folate, Magnesium Manganese, Potassium, Vitamin B6, Vitamin C, Vitamin K1

White fruits and vegetables have even been linked to lowering the risk of a stroke. In 2021, researchers at Wageningen University in The Netherlands found that a 25g a day increase in white fruits and vegetables were linked with a 9% lower risk of a stroke after examining 20,000 adults with an average age of 41 years old.

HEALTHY PROTEIN

As we mentioned in Chapter 7, protein is the building material that the body uses to construct every part of you. Protein is the fundamental building block of organs, muscle, skin and hormones. We need protein to help maintain and repair tissues (children need it for growth), send messages around the body, balance fluid levels, bolster immune health, and provide energy. There are more than 10,000 types of proteins in your body, and they are all made up of chains of amino acids. Out of the twenty amino acids that make up these proteins, nine cannot be made by the body. These are called essential amino acids and must be obtained from the foods we eat.

The UDS National Academy of Medicine recommends that adults consume a minimum of 0.8 g of protein for every kilogram of body weight. In other words, an individual weighing 70 kg (approximately 155 lb) would require 56 g of protein per day. However, protein intake can increase to up to 2 g per kilogram for more active individuals, depending on the activity. For example, a bodybuilder would consume a far higher protein content than a golfer. A diet that is high in protein may help to lower blood pressure, as well as fight conditions such as type 2 diabetes. Plus, protein helps you to stay fuller for longer, so can also help with appetite control.

The Best Protein Sources

While protein is a critical part of a healthy diet, many protein foods are high in calories and fat. It is important, therefore, that you make the right protein choices. Here are the ten top proteins that you should include on your plate:

1. White Fleshed Fish - white fish is extremely lean, with most varieties providing less than 3 grams of fat for a 100 g serving. That 100 g will also provide you with 20-25 g of protein. You should aim for two portions of fish per week.

2. Plain Greek Yogurt - a 170 g serving will provide 15-20 g of protein. Twice as much as you will get from regular yogurt!

3. Beans, Peas and Lentils - a 100 g serving of any of these legumes will average 8 g of protein and provide lots of fiber.

4. Skinless, white meat poultry - a 100 g serving of white meat chicken will provide 30 g of protein.

5. Low fat cottage cheese - a half cup of low-fat cottage cheese will provide 13 g of protein and just 2.5 g of fat.

6. Tofu - tofu is one of the very plant-based sources of all 11 essential amino acids. An 85 g serving will provide you with 7 g of protein.

7. Lean Beef - lean cuts of beef contain less than 10 g of fat. A 100 g lean cooked hamburger will provide you with 26 g of protein.

8. Low Fat Milk - A glass of 1% low-fat milk contains 8 g of protein and about 100 calories.

9. Eggs - an average-sized egg will provide 6 g of protein and 48 calories.

10. Pork Loin - pork tenderloin is the leanest cut of pork, providing 26 g of protein, 143 calories and 3.5 g of fat for every 100 g serving.

HEALTHY OILS

Healthy oils – suggested as an added extra by the Healthy Eating Plate – are a source of dietary fat. Dietary fat is a vital component of a healthy, balanced nutrition plan. There is a common belief that saturated fats are bad and unsaturated fats are good. However, good health requires a balance of fatty acids, including saturated fats. As saturated fats primarily come from animal sources, your quota of these will come from your 'Healthy Protein' section of the food plate. A good rule of thumb when it comes to saturated fat is that:

- Men should have no more than 30 grams of saturated fat daily
- Women should have no more than 20 grams of saturated fat daily

The majority of unsaturated fats, on the other hand, come from vegetable and plant sources. They come under two subcategories:

- Monounsaturated fats

- Polyunsaturated fats

Monounsaturated fats have the ability to reduce blood cholesterol levels and insulin levels. The best food sources of monounsaturated fats to include on your food plate are:

- Olives and olive oil
- Nuts and nut oils (e.g. coconut oil, peanut oil)
- Avocado
- Canola Oil

Unsaturated fats are also present in some types of fish, and are known as **omega-3 fatty acids**. Omega-3 fatty acids and other nutrients in fish may benefit heart health and reduce the risk of dying of heart disease. One of your recommended two portions of fish per week should be oily fish.

A good rule of thumb to follow when selecting healthy oils and fats is to avoid foods that are highly processed and that contain ingredients that you cannot even pronounce. Foods such as French Fries (and other deep-fried foods), crackers and baked goods are examples of foods that contain what are known as trans-fats. These fats are modified through the process of hydrogenation to preserve shelf life.

GUIDELINES ON SUGAR AND SALT

Finally, we need to talk about salt (sodium) and sugar.

High levels of sodium in the blood can contribute to inflammation. Over time, this can put you at serious risk of health issues such as high blood pressure, stroke, heart and kidney failure, and some cancers.

Despite this, salt is an important nutrient for the human body, so it is important that you don't cut it out completely! Instead, adults should aim to eat no more than 6 g of salt daily.

Consuming too much sugar, on the other hand, can lead to obesity, which itself is a risk factor for diabetes and heart disease. Excessive sugar in the diet can also lead to tooth decay. Current guidelines state that:

- No more than 5 percent of daily calories should come from sugar.
- Adults should have no more than 30 g of sugar daily (7 sugar cubes).

EATING IN MODERATION

There is no such thing as good or bad food. There are most definitely foods that you should eat more often than others. Those are the ones that I've highlighted in the preceding sections. That doesn't mean that foods that are not on those lists are forbidden. Instead, they should be enjoyed occasionally. You will actually find when you limit them to occasional or treat time snacks, you will enjoy them a whole lot more.

Here are a dozen foods you should eat in moderation:

- French Fries
- Burgers
- Donuts
- Pizza
- Biscuits
- Ice Cream
- Alcohol
- Chocolate
- Snack Bars
- Potato Chips

RECAP OF KEY RECOMMENDATIONS:

1. The majority of your plate should be made up of plants. Eat at least 30 portions of a variety of plant-based foods (wholegrains, fruit and vegetables) every week.
2. Eat lots of beans, pulses, fish, eggs, meat and

other proteins (including 2 portions of fish every week, one of which should be oily).

3. Drink 6-8 cups/glasses of fluid a day, avoiding sugary drinks and alcohol. You will need more water if you exercise.

4. Foods high in saturated and/ or trans-fats, salt and sugar should be consumed in small amounts infrequently (no more than 6 g of salt, and 30 g of sugar on a daily basis).

PORTION SIZES

When it comes to how much food to actually fit on your plate per meal, it really does depend on a number of factors such as age, metabolism and physical activity. We're all different shapes and sizes and men and women have different recommended calorie intakes per day. Some of us prefer a bigger breakfast and a small dinner and vice versa.

We've already learned that smaller 9-inch plates and avoiding seconds will help reduce portion sizes but let's now look at dividing our daily calories up into meals, drinks and snacks. It's generally advised to eat your larger meals earlier in the day, so we'll go on that premise.

A woman's daily calorie intake in 2000, so let's break that down.

- Breakfast is 500 calories
- Lunch is 500 calories
- Dinner is 400 calories
- 400ml glass of 2% fat milk is 200 calories
- Snack number 1 is 200 calories.
- Snack number 2 is 200 calories
- 8 glasses of water is zero calories

A man's daily calorie intake is 2500, so as a man, you simply have an extra 500 calories per day to play around with.

This is just an example but I wouldn't recommend obsessing about calories, just as I do not recommend obsessing about the bathroom scales. There is give or take and you might need to eat more if you have been doing heavy resistance training or intense cardio that day. Keeping track of your calories is important but remember the key here is to follow the guidance in chapters 5 and 6, be mindful about your food, listen to your body and know when you are full.

SUMMARY

From this chapter, we really start to gain practical knowledge of what types of food we should eat. We can now start to proportion our meals in terms of macronutrients, knowing what our daily plate should look like. We also have vital micronutrient information to hand in order to put into practice and to go out to the grocery store and fill your fridge and pantry with color and diversity. As you can see there are dozens of fruits and vegetables that you can choose from. Be bold and experimental with your choices as only positive health benefits will come from a wide range of micronutrients. In our next chapter, we'll delve into a whole load of food tips as well as recipes for each daily meal to help get you started on your new and healthy lifestyle. We're almost there, so let's keep going!

9

CHANGES TO MAKE IN MEALS, SNACKS AND DESSERTS

"Food may be essential as fuel for the body, but GOOD food is fuel for the soul"

— MALCOLM FORBES

I n our penultimate chapter, I reveal a range of simple ideas, suggestions and recipes that you can make immediately to improve your nutrition and improve your health. I'll divide them into sections based on the traditional three main meals of the day.

BREAKFAST

Here are ten tips to make every-day breakfasts healthier:

- Replace bacon rashes with medallions or turkey bacon. Or just one rash of regular bacon. Avoid streaky bacon as it is higher in fat.
- If you love sausages like most people do, cut down to just one sausage, find low-fat lean pork sausages, or use chicken or veggie ones.
- Try cauliflower hash browns instead of potato.
- Poach your eggs or use extra egg whites in your scrambled eggs or omelet for extra protein—no more than two yolks per person.
- Use semi skimmed or skimmed milk for oatmeal/porridge. There are also other great alternatives such as oat and almond milk.
- Change to wholemeal bread instead of white.
- Add in some vegetables or fruit. For example: grilled tomato, asparagus and tender stem broccoli are amazing with poached eggs.
- Add walnuts and a sprinkling of cinnamon to oatmeal.
- Include protein in the form of Greek yogurt.
- Blend up a breakfast smoothie, combining fruit, juice, yogurt, wheat germ, tofu and berries.

5 GREAT BREAKFAST RECIPE IDEAS

Banana Pancakes

Dry Ingredients

- 1.5 cups white whole wheat flour
- 1.5 teaspoons baking powder
- 1/2 teaspoon ground cinnamon
- 1/8 teaspoon salt

Wet Ingredients

- 2 medium bananas, mashed (~1 cup puree)
- 2 large eggs
- 1 teaspoon vanilla extract
- 1 cup unsweetened almond milk
- 3 tablespoons melted coconut oil
- Drizzle of honey (optional)

Method

1. First, combine dry ingredients in a medium bowl and set aside.
2. Mash bananas in a large bowl until there are only a few lumps and they are pureed. Then, add in eggs, vanilla, and almond milk and whisk until smooth.

3. Slowly add dry ingredients to wet and mix to combine. Finally, add in melted coconut oil and mix until smooth. Your batter should be thick.
4. Heat a non-stick pan over medium heat. Spray with coconut oil cooking spray. When the oil is hot, scoop about 1/3 cup of the batter onto your pan and cook for 2-3 minutes on each side, flipping when the bubbles start to form in the center of the pancakes.
5. Repeat until all batter is gone.
6. Top with sliced banana and honey.

Low Carb Breakfast Burritos

Ingredients

- 2 large eggs
- 1 tbsp. Skimmed milk
- 1 tbsp. Freshly chopped chives
- Sprinkle of salt
- Freshly ground black pepper
- 1 tbsp. Butter
- 2 slices cooked bacon
- 1/2 c. Black beans
- 1 avocado, thinly sliced
- 1/2 c. shredded cheddar
- Salsa, for serving

Method

1. In a small bowl, whisk together eggs, milk, and chives, and season with salt and pepper.
2. In a large non-stick skillet, melt butter. Once the pan is completely coated, add the egg mixture. Tilt pan back and forth to make sure it's completely coated, then let cook, 2 minutes. Once you can move the egg back and forth, carefully flip and cook 2 minutes more.
3. Transfer to a plate and top with bacon, black beans, avocado, cheddar, and salsa. Roll up into a burrito and serve.

Smoked Salmon and Poached Egg with Green Vegetables

Ingredients

- 50g smoked salmon
- 2 medium eggs
- 4 sticks of asparagus
- 4 sticks tender stem broccoli
- 1/4 tsp. Salt
- 1/4 tsp. Black pepper
- 30-40 mg. White wine vinegar
- ¼ squeezed lemon

Method

1. Turn your grill to a medium-high heat and place the asparagus and broccoli under the grill for 5 minutes, turning half way.
2. Bring a saucepan of water and the white wine vinegar to medium heat so it's lightly bubbling.
3. Crack the 2 eggs and poach for 2 – 2 ½ minutes. Meanwhile, place the salmon on the plate.
4. Place the eggs on some kitchen paper to soak up any remaining water.
5. Serve eggs and vegetables on the plate. Squeeze the lemon and season according to taste.

Easy Kale Feta Egg Toast

Ingredients

- 2 slices English muffin bread, sourdough bread, multigrain bread, or English muffin, for serving
- 3 teaspoons olive oil divided
- 3 cups chopped kale stems removed
- 1 teaspoon minced garlic (2 cloves)
- 1/8 teaspoon salt plus additional for seasoning
- 1/8 teaspoon pepper plus additional for seasoning
- 1/8 teaspoon red pepper flakes

- 2 large eggs
- 2 ounces feta cheese crumbled

Method

1. Toast bread in a toaster, toaster oven, or beneath a broiler. Set aside.
2. Heat 2 teaspoons of olive oil in a large skillet on medium heat. Add the kale, stir to coat, then cook, occasionally stirring, until the kale begins to soften, about 5 minutes.
3. Add the garlic, ⅛ teaspoon salt, ⅛ teaspoon pepper, and red pepper flakes. Stir and cook for 1 additional minute. Remove from heat, stir in the feta cheese, then cover to keep warm.
4. In a small skillet, heat the remaining teaspoon of olive oil over medium. Gently crack eggs into skillet and sprinkle with a little extra salt and pepper.
5. Cook until the whites are nearly set, about 1 minute. Cover skillet, remove from heat and let stand until whites are set but yolks are still soft, about 3 minutes.
6. To serve: Place half of the kale on top of each toast, then top with a fried egg. Serve immediately.

Frittatas

Ingredients

- ¼ c. Spinach
- ¼ c. Chopped onion
- ¼ c. Chopped peppers
- 1 tomato sliced
- 2 eggs
- ¼ c. Crumbled feta
- Salt and pepper to season
- 1 tbsp. Olive oil
- 2 slices of wholemeal toast
- Watercress

Method

1. Wisk the 2 eggs in a bowl with a splash of milk if desired and add salt and pepper to taste. Chop the tomato into thin slices.
2. Heat the olive oil in a frying pan on a medium-high heat and heat your grill to a high temperature.
3. Add the onions and peppers to the pan for 3 minutes then the spinach for 1 more minute.
4. Add the eggs and make sure they cover the whole frying pan.

5. Place the tomato slices on top and sprinkle the feta.
6. Put toast on in the toaster and heat the frittata on the pan for 2 minutes on a medium heat.
7. Place the frying pan under the grill for 2 minutes.
8. Butter the toast, place the water cress on the side.
9. Fold the Frittata in half if desired and serve.

5 GREAT LUNCH IDEAS

Easy Healthy Salad Sandwich

Ingredients

For the herb mayo

- 1/3 cup mayonnaise
- ¼ cup fresh herbs of your choice (basil, parsley, chives)
- a squeeze of lemon juice
- salt and pepper to taste

For the sandwich

- 2 slices whole-grain bread
- sliced tomato

- sliced cucumber
- sliced red onion
- julienned carrot
- lettuce / arugula / baby spinach
- sliced cheese (optional)

Method

1. Combine all the mayo ingredients and blend with an immersion blender until smooth. Alternatively, use a blender or food processor.
2. To assemble the sandwich, spread a generous dollop of the mayo onto each slice of bread and top with the vegetables and cheese. Sandwich, slice and serve.

Spiced Lentil & Butternut Squash Soup

Ingredients

- 2 tbsp olive oil
- 2 onions, finely chopped
- 2 garlic cloves, crushed
- ¼ tsp hot chili powder
- 1 tbsp ras el hanout
- 1 butternut squash, peeled and cut into 2cm pieces
- 100g red lentils

- 1liter hot vegetable stock
- 1 small bunch coriander, leaves chopped, plus extra to serve
- Natural yogurt, to serve

Method

1. Heat the oil in a large flameproof casserole dish or saucepan over medium-high heat. Fry the onions with a pinch of salt for 7 mins, or until softened and just caramelized. Add the garlic, chili and ras el hanout, and cook for 1 min more.
2. Stir in the squash and lentils. Pour over the stock and season to taste. Bring to the boil, then reduce the heat to a simmer and cook, cover for 25 mins or until the squash is soft.
3. Blitz the soup with a stick blender until smooth, then season to taste. To freeze, leave to cool completely and transfer to large freezer-proof bags.
4. Stir in the coriander leaves and ladle the soup into bowls. Serve topped with the dukkah, yogurt and extra coriander leaves.

Bright and Spicy Shrimp Noodle Salad

Ingredients

- ⅓ cup fresh lime juice
- 2 tsp. honey
- 1 serrano chile, very thinly sliced
- 1 inch piece of ginger, peeled, finely grated
- 1 garlic clove, finely grated
- 1 Tbsp plus 1½ tsp fish sauce
- 4 Tbsp. extra-virgin olive oil
- Salt
- 1 lb. large shrimp (preferably wild), peeled, deveined
- 6 oz. bean thread (cellophane or glass) noodles
- 1 cucumber, halved lengthwise, thinly sliced crosswise
- ½ cup salted, roasted peanuts, crushed
- 1 cup basil leaves

Method

1. Stir lime juice and honey in a small bowl until honey dissolves. Mix in chile, ginger, garlic, fish sauce, and 3 Tbsp of oil; season dressing with salt.
2. Toss shrimp and 2 Tbsp of dressing in a medium bowl to coat; let sit for 10 minutes.

3. Meanwhile, cook noodles according to package directions. Drain and add to the bowl with remaining dressing along with cucumber and ¼ cup peanuts; toss well.

4. Heat remaining 1 Tbsp of oil in a large nonstick skillet over medium-high. Pour off any liquid from shrimp and pat dry; season all over with salt. Cook shrimp, occasionally tossing, until browned and bright pink, about 5 minutes. Transfer to a bowl with noodles, add basil and toss well to combine.

5. Divide noodle salad among bowls and top with remaining peanuts.

Lemony Salmon and Spiced Chickpeas

Ingredients

- 1 lemon, thinly sliced, seeds removed
- ½ cup extra-virgin olive oil, plus more for drizzling
- 1½-lb. salmon fillet, preferably skin-on
- ½ tsp. Salt
- Freshly ground black pepper
- 15-oz. can chickpeas, rinsed, patted dry
- 1 garlic clove, finely chopped
- 2 tsp. za'atar
- 1 tsp. fresh lemon juice

- 4 cups baby arugula or baby spinach
- 4 radishes, trimmed, thinly sliced
- Flaky sea salt

Method

1. Place a rack in the lower third of the oven; preheat to 300°. Toss lemon slices in a large bowl with a drizzle of oil. Arrange slices in an even layer on a rimmed baking sheet. Set salmon on lemons. Season salmon all over with salt and pepper, then drizzle and rub with some oil. Roast until the salmon is just barely opaque in the middle, 12–17 minutes, depending on thickness. If you like your salmon well-done, cook it a few minutes longer, but keep in mind that you risk the chance it will dry out. Let salmon cool, then flake into medium-size pieces with a fork.

2. Meanwhile, bring chickpeas, garlic, za'atar, and remaining ½ cup oil to a bare simmer in a small skillet over medium-low heat. Cook, stirring occasionally and reducing heat if needed, 10 minutes. Stir in ½ tsp of salt (less if your za'atar is salty) and remove skillet from heat.

3. Using a slotted spoon, transfer chickpeas to a medium bowl, leaving oil behind. Whisk lemon

juice into oil; taste dressing and season with more salt and a few grinds of pepper if needed.

4. Toss arugula in a large bowl with 1 tsp of dressing. Divide among bowls along with radishes, chickpeas, and salmon (and lemons if desired); drizzle with more dressing. Sprinkle it with sea salt and more pepper.

Bean Salad Bowl with Asian Glaze

Ingredients

For the salad

- Broad beans
- Green beans
- Red onion
- Cherry tomatoes
- Cucumber
- Mixed peppers
- Leafy greens like spinach, rocket, watercress or lettuce
- Quinoa
- Pre-cooked shrimp, sliced chicken or steak (optional)

For the Asian glaze (serves 4, so save some in the fridge for another meal)

- 3 cloves chopped garlic
- 1 inch block of ginger, chopped
- ¼ cup. honey
- ¼ cup of soy sauce
- 3 tablespoons of rice vinegar
- 2 tablespoons hoisin sauce
- 1 tablespoon sesame oil
- ½ teaspoon of chilli flakes (optional for spice)

Method

1. Lightly boil the broad and green beans for 3 minutes, then run them under cold water
2. In a pan, lightly boil the quinoa, usually about 15 mins (check the packaging for cooking time)
3. Chop the onion, tomato and cucumber
4. If desired, grill your chicken breast or steak of choice, then cut into slices. Let it cool down
5. Add the sauce ingredients into a pan and gently boil for 5 minutes. Keep stirring to avoid it sticking to the pan. Let it cool down
6. Add the leafy greens, beans and all other veg into a bowl
7. Once the quinoa is done, let it cool down and add to the bowl
8. Add your chicken, steak or pre-cooked cold shrimp on top, then add the glaze

DINNER

My Top 22 Tips

1. Make a roast chicken for dinner, use the remaining meat for chicken salads and sandwiches, and boil the bones to make stock for healthy soups.
2. Use turkey thigh or breast mince (thigh is much tastier) instead of red meat mince like beef or lamb.
3. Make mash from either sweet potato or cannellini beans rather than white potato.
4. If you hate broccoli, try grilled or pan-fried tender stem broccoli to help introduce you to the flavor.
5. Use seasonings, herbs and spices for your meat and fish rather than sauces.
6. Use things like lemon, lime, wine, olive oils for lighter dressings rather than creamy sauces.
7. Use crème fresh instead of cream for sauces and desserts.
8. Find a low sugar protein bar with fiber that you really like or better yet make your own, and always have one on you as a healthier snack instead of a candy bar.
9. Use Greek yogurt (full fat) with a drizzle of

honey and fruit rather than store-bought yogurt or unhealthy desserts.

10. Freeze your bread so you don't need to rush using it before the use-by date.

11. Buy a juicer and make your own fresh fruit juice instead of added sugar fruit juice from the shops.

12. Buy a Nutribullet and make your own fruit and veg smoothies or protein shakes. Add whole oats for extra fiber.

13. Learn to poach an egg as it's quick and healthy.

14. If you're craving something fizzy, drink sparkling mineral water with no added sugar squash instead of high sugary sodas.

15. Half and half Courgette aka Zucchini with pasta to avoid meals like bolognaise or carbonara being too high in carb.

16. Try to get used to brown rice and pasta over time. Brown basmati is nicer, so start with that.

17. Instead of salted crisps as snacks, eat nuts. Unsalted almonds, walnuts, brazil and cashew are high in nutrition.

18. When making stir fry meals, use it as an opportunity to add in as much vegetables as possible. Buy a good stir fry veg mix, add in green beans, sugar snap peas, broccoli, spring greens...the list goes on and on! Mix up your

meat or fish, i.e. One week pork, the next week shrimp, the next week vegetables only!

19. Try to avoid using packaged stir fry sauces and make your own. Personally, ginger, chilli, lemon and lime juice, a splash of soy sauce, and a splash of white wine work great!

20. Replace the frying pan with your grill or an air fryer. For example, Grilled bacon, pork chops, chicken etc. You can boil your potatoes then put them in the air fryer for 5-10 minutes and they will crispen up without using all that oil in a frying pan. This also works well with steak!

21. If you hate or simply don't have time to always chop up vegetables, buy frozen chopped vegetables like onions and peppers to save time and stress.

22. Cook healthy bulk meals and portion them up straight away into Tupperware so you have extra meals for lunches or dinners. This will also prevent you from having seconds after dinner.

5 GREAT DINNER IDEAS

Spanish Chicken

Ingredients

- 4 boneless skinless chicken breasts - OR 6 chicken thighs
- 3 tablespoons vegetable or canola oil
- 1 cup uncooked brown basmati rice
- 2 ¼ cups low salt chicken broth
- 1 lemon
- chopped cilantro or parsley - for garnish
- Green vegetables like broccoli, sugar snap peas, spring greens

For the Spanish Mix Seasoning

- 2 teaspoons smoked paprika
- 1 teaspoon garlic powder
- 1 teaspoon salt
- 1 teaspoon ground cumin
- 1 teaspoon chili powder
- 1 teaspoon coriander
- ¼ teaspoon Italian seasoning

Method

1. In a small bowl, whisk together all ingredients for the Spanish seasoning mix. Divide in half and set aside. Cut the lemon in half, then thinly slice one half - for garnish - and reserve the other half for juicing later in the recipe.

2. Place chicken in a medium bowl. Drizzle with 2 tablespoons of oil, then toss to coat well. Use half of the prepared seasoning mix to rub on both sides of each piece of chicken.

3. Drizzle a large skillet with the remaining 1 tablespoon of oil and bring to medium heat. Cook chicken for 2-3 minutes on each side until browned. Transfer to a plate. (It won't be cooked through at this point).

4. Add rice, chicken broth, juice from 1/2 of the lemon, and remaining seasoning mix and stir to combine. Return the chicken to the pan on top of the rice. Cover and cook for 20-25 minutes until liquid is absorbed, rice is tender, and chicken is cooked through.

5. Steam the extra vegetables of choice according to the packet guidelines.

6. Garnish with lemon slices and freshly chopped cilantro or parsley and serve immediately.

Turkey Mince Bolognaise with Zucchini and Extra Vegetables

Ingredients

- 500g turkey thigh mince
- Half an onion
- 1 green pepper
- 1 large carrot
- 1 stick of celery
- 1 zucchini aka courgette
- 1 ½ tins chopped tomato
- 1 small lemon (juice)
- Italian herbs
- Fresh basil
- 1 beef stockpot
- 3 cloves of garlic
- Salt and pepper
- Olive oil
- Splash of red wine
- Wholemeal spaghetti
- A light sprinkle of grated cheese (if desired)

Method

1. Chop the onions, peppers, carrots and celery into small pieces.

2. Heat the oil in a large pan or wok on a medium-high heat.

3. Add the onions, peppers, carrots and celery into the pan and fry for 2-3 minutes.

4. Add the mince and cook till brown. Meanwhile, chop the garlic into small pieces.

5. Boil the water for the pasta and add a pinch of salt.

6. Add the tomatoes, wine, lemon juice, Italian herbs, stockpot, salt, pepper and garlic into the pan and simmer on a medium heat for 20 minutes.

7. Cook the pasta on the hob for 8-10 minutes.

8. If you have a spiralizer, prepare the zucchini. You do not need to cook the zucchini. Place the spaghetti and zucchini into a bowl (half and half), then the sauce on top.

9. Grate the cheese and place the fresh basil on top.

Shrimp & Broccoli

Ingredients

- 1 pound large shrimp, deveined (peeled or unpeeled)
- 1 1/2 pounds broccoli (heads and stems)
- 1 small white onion

- 2 tablespoons rice vinegar
- 4 tablespoons soy sauce
- ½ tablespoon chili garlic sauce (optional)
- 2 tablespoons sesame oil
- ¼ teaspoon salt
- Sesame seeds, for garnish
- Thinly sliced green onion for garnish (optional)
- To serve: rice or noodles

Method

1. If frozen, thaw the shrimp according to the package instructions or the notes above.
2. Chop the broccoli into small bite-sized pieces. Cut the onion into wide slices.
3. In a measuring cup, stir together the rice vinegar, soy sauce, and chili garlic sauce.
4. If serving with rice, remember to allow time for the rice to cook. Usually around 10 minutes for white and 20 - 25 minutes for brown. If serving with noodles, usually allow 3- 5 minutes. Check all packaging first to get your timing right.
5. In a large skillet or wok, heat the sesame oil over medium-high heat. Add the broccoli, onion and salt and cook for 5 to 6 minutes until fork-tender, stirring occasionally. Add the

shrimp and cook for 3 to 4 minutes, stirring frequently.

6. When the shrimp is just about opaque, add the sauce mixture and cook for 1 minute. Remove from the heat. Serve with sesame seeds.

Grilled Chicken with Charred Pineapple Salad

Ingredients

- 1 teaspoon dried oregano
- Olive oil
- 2 x 150 g free-range chicken breasts
- 150 g quinoa
- 50 g white cabbage
- 1 large handful of salad leaves
- ¼ of a pineapple
- 50 g natural Greek yogurt
- 1 fresh red chili

Dressing

- ½ an avocado
- ½ a bunch of fresh coriander, (15g)
- 2 tablespoons pickled jalapeños
- 2 limes

Method

1. Combine the oregano in a bowl with 1 to 2 tablespoons of oil, then season with sea salt and black pepper.

2. Use a sharp knife to slice into the chicken breasts, then open each one out flat like a book to butterfly. Place in the bowl with the herby oil, turning until well coated, then leave to one side.

3. Cook the quinoa according to the packet instructions, then drain and set aside.

4. For the dressing, peel and destone the avocado half, then scoop the flesh into a blender. Add half the coriander (stalks and all) and the jalapeños, along with a splash of the pickling liquid and the juice of 1½ limes. Blitz until smooth, adding a splash of oil if needed. Stir through the quinoa.

5. Finely shred the cabbage, pick the remaining coriander leaves, then toss with the salad leaves.

6. Place a griddle pan over high heat. Peel the pineapple, remove and discard any core, then chop into 4. Place on the hot griddle pan for a few minutes on each side, or until charred, and transfer to a chopping board. In the same pan, griddle the chicken for 5 minutes on each side,

or until charred and cooked through, then remove from the pan and leave to rest on the board for a few minutes.

7. Chop the griddled pineapple into bite-sized chunks, then slice the chicken into thin strips. Deseed and finely chop the chili.

8. Divide the yogurt between four plates, then top with the chicken, adding the pineapple on one side and the dressed quinoa on the other. Toss the leaves and cabbage with the juice of the remaining lime half and a little salt and pepper, plus the chopped chili. Divide between the plates, then serve.

Steak Dijon

Ingredients

- 4 medium sweet potatoes
- 2 steaks of choice
- 1 tbsp. canola oil
- 1 medium onion
- 1 c. low salt chicken broth
- 2 tbsp. finely chopped fresh dill
- 1 tbsp. Dijon mustard
- 1 lb. green beans

Method

1. Peel the Sweet potatoes then, in a pan of boiling water, carefully add the potatoes and slow boil them on medium-high heat until soft. Drain well.
2. Meanwhile, in a 12-inch skillet, heat oil on medium-high. Sprinkle steaks with 1/4 teaspoon each salt and pepper; cook 2 to 3 minutes per side on medium-high heat or until the desired doneness. Transfer to a cutting board and cover with foil.
3. In the same skillet, cook the onion for 2 minutes, stirring. Stir in broth; heat to simmering. Simmer for 5 minutes. Whisk in dill, mustard, and 1/4 teaspoon pepper.
4. Steam the green beans as directed on the packet. Usually 3-4 minutes.
5. Mash sweet potatoes. You will not need any butter, milk, cheese or salt.
6. Slice steak; serve with potatoes, green beans, and sauce.

10 HEALTHIER DESSERT OPTIONS

1. Fruit
2. Chia Pudding

3. Greek Yogurt
4. Peanut Butter and Banana Ice Cream
5. Low Sugar Popsicles
6. Nut Butter
7. Baked Pears or Apples
8. Chocolate Dipped Banana Bites
9. DIY Chocolate Truffles
10. Baked Sweet Potatoes

MAKE YOUR OWN PROTEIN BARS

Protein bars provide a convenient on-the-go protein source. However, store-bought bars are both expensive and liable to contain fillers, flavorings and preservatives. You can and should make your own no-bake protein bars.

Protein Nut Bar Recipe

Ingredients

- 2 1/2 cups (250 g) old-fashioned certified gluten-free rolled oats (if gluten-free isn't necessary, use any oats)
- 1 1/2 scoops (54 g) gluten-free protein powder (I like Vega essentials chocolate flavor protein powder, but you can use whey protein or your favorite protein powder (vanilla or chocolate))

- 1/2 cup (40 g) unsweetened cocoa powder (natural or Dutch-processed) (can replace with more protein powder)
- 3/4 cup (192 g) smooth natural nut butter (I have used peanut butter, almond butter and cashew butter—all work well)
- 1/4 cup (84 g) pure maple syrup
- 1/4 teaspoon salt
- 1/4 cup (2 fluid ounces) milk (any kind), plus more as necessary
- 3 ounces unsweetened chocolate, chopped and melted (can replace with 2 tablespoons more nut butter + 1 tablespoon pure maple syrup)
- 8 ounces bittersweet chocolate, chopped and melted (optional, for coating)

Method

1. Line an 8-inch square baking pan or standard 9-inch x 5-inch loaf pan with unbleached parchment paper and set it aside.
2. To make the date version, place the oats in a food processor fitted with the steel blade and process until ground into flour. Add the protein powder, dates, maple syrup, vanilla, salt, 1/4 cup milk and (optional) melted unsweetened chocolate. Process until the mixture is well-

combined and is tacky (but not sticky) to the touch. Add more milk by the teaspoonful and process, only as necessary for the mixture to reach the proper consistency. If you opt not to use the melted unsweetened chocolate, you will have to add more milk, and the bars will not hold together as firmly when shaped.

3. Transfer the mixture to the prepared pan and press firmly into an even layer, smoothing the top as much as possible. Cover with parchment and place in the refrigerator or freezer to chill until firm (about 1 hour in the refrigerator, or 20 minutes in the freezer). Remove the bars from the pan and slice them into 10 or 12 equal-sized rectangular bars. Dip in the optional melted bittersweet chocolate to coat and allow to sit at room temperature until set. Store the bars in a sealed container in the refrigerator.

4. To make the nut butter version, place the oats in a food processor fitted with the steel blade and process until ground into flour. Add the protein powder, cocoa powder (or more protein powder), nut butter, maple syrup, salt, 1/4 cup milk and melted unsweetened chocolate (or more nut butter and maple syrup). Process until the mixture is well-combined and is tacky (but

not sticky) to the touch. Add more milk by the teaspoonful and process, only as necessary for the mixture to reach the proper consistency.

5. Transfer the mixture to the prepared pan and press firmly into an even layer, smoothing the top as much as possible. Cover with parchment and place in the refrigerator or freezer to chill until firm (about 1 hour in the refrigerator, or 20 minutes in the freezer). Remove the bars from the pan and slice into 10 or 12 equal-sized rectangular bars. Dip in the optional melted bittersweet chocolate to coat or simply drizzle some melted chocolate over the top, and allow to sit at room temperature until set. Wrap the bars individually in waxed paper, and store in the refrigerator.

THE SMOOTHIE SOLUTION

Getting into the Smoothie habit will make it a whole lot easier for you to provide your body with the nutrients it needs to thrive.

Here are 5 reasons why you should embrace the smoothie habit . . .

Lowered Cholesterol

High levels of low-density lipoprotein (LDL) cholesterol have been associated with all manner of cardiac
problems. Getting into the smoothie habit will help to
lower your LDL cholesterol levels. If you replace a
breakfast of bacon, eggs and toast with a fruit-filled
smoothie, you will automatically cut back your LDL
cholesterol intake. On top of that, the fruits that are
included in your smoothies are filled with phytochemicals, antioxidants and other properties that reduce LDL
cholesterol. The best fruits to include to bring down
your LDL cholesterol levels are apples, blueberries,
strawberries, avocados, grapes and citrus fruits.

Immunity-Boosting

The vitamins, minerals, phytochemicals and antioxidants that are in smoothies will boost your immunity.
This will better ward off colds, flu and viruses. Focus
on citrus juices to get the most immunity-boosting
benefit from your smoothies.

Heart Health

We have already mentioned how smoothies can help
lower LDL cholesterol levels. But that's not the only
way they benefit your heart health. Including citrus
fruits in your smoothies will provide you with potassium and folate. Potassium helps to keep your blood

pressure levels in check, while folate helps to produce healthy blood cells.

Improves Digestion

When you drink a fruit-infused smoothie, you will be taking in between 2 and 7 grams of fiber. This will help to keep your digestive system functioning with maximum efficiency. When you take your fruits in the form of a smoothie, the process of digestion is much easier because the fruits are already partially broken down. This helps to eliminate such digestive problems as gas, bloating and indigestion that many people experience when they eat fruit.

Convenience

Let's face it – our lives are busy. Finding the time to prepare a proper dinner meal is challenging enough. Preparing several nutritionally balanced meals over the course of your day can be totally overwhelming. But when you replace one of those meals with a super delicious, quick-to-prepare smoothie, suddenly things become way more manageable.

3 GREAT SMOOTHIE RECIPES

Berry Explosion

Ingredients

- 1 x Scoop of Strawberry Protein Powder
- 1/2 cup of Blueberries
- ½ cup of raspberries
- 4 strawberries
- 1 x Cup of Coconut Milk
- 2-3 Ice Cubes

Method

1. Place the berries in your blender
2. Add 1 cup of unsweetened Coconut Milk
3. Add 2-3 Ice cubes
4. Add the Strawberry Protein Powder
5. Blend all ingredients for 30-45 sec

Green Power Cleansing Juice

Ingredients

- 2 x Big kale leaves
- 1/2 Cup x baby spinach leaves
- 1 x chopped cucumber

- 1 x apple roughly chopped
- 1 x Lemon peeled
- 1⁄2 Bunch mint
- Option to add ginger

Method

1. Juice all ingredients together in a juicer and pour over ice if desired.

Tropical Protein Heaven

Ingredients

1. 1 x cup coconut milk
2. 1/2 x banana
3. 1/2 cup x chopped pineapple
4. 1/2 cup x chopped mango
5. 2 scoops x Vanilla Protein Powder
6. crushed ice

Method

1. Blend all ingredients and pour over ice.

Many recipes in this chapter are courtesy of:

www.wellplated.com

www.feastingathome.com

www.acouplecooks.com

www.jamieoliver.com

www.delish.com

https://glutenfreeonashoestring.com

https://www.modernhoney.com

https://drivemehungry.com/sweet-and-tangy-sticky-soy-glaze/

SUMMARY

There are literally millions of food ideas, tips and recipes out there. We all have different tastes and dietary requirements, some of which require very specific attention to detail. For most of you reading this chapter, you will be able to take the majority of these recipes and put them into practice. This is also a great opportunity to expand your food knowledge as there's a whole new world out there of amazing chefs and recipe books. You could even take it a step further and sign up to either weekly cooking classes or a one-off weekend masterclass. The options are all out there for you so take advantage of them! Remember, food is a gift. It's meant to be appreciated, respected but most importantly embraced and enjoyed!

CONCLUSION

"Success is not final. Failure is not fatal. It is the courage to continue that counts"

— SIR WINSTON CHURCHILL

Over the course of our journey together, we have charted a course toward new, better, healthier eating habits that you can easily adopt and ingrain into your lifestyle. In the process, you have discovered how to finally break the bad habits that have been enslaving you to a way of eating that you've known is no good but been powerless to do anything about. Well, now you have the power!

How have we done it?

At the outset, I laid out our template for success. It was based on the following 3 fundamental steps:

Step 1 – Identifying habits throughout our lives and understanding why these have manifested.

Step 2 – Change our mindset and learn how to break those habits through self-reflection, honesty and mindful eating techniques.

Step 3 – Implement practical knowledge solutions to provide you with a detailed basic education in nutrition, along with valuable tips and meal ideas.

Let's now review the key takeaways under each of these steps . . .

STEP ONE: IDENTIFYING HABITS

During our formative years, we develop the habits that will drive your nutritional future. The habits are a combination of prenatal nutrition, cultural differences, food company advertising, parental example, social media influences, peer pressure, and societal pressures.

What We've Learnt About Ourselves

1. Ageing. As we age, our bodies undergo the following detrimental changes . . .

- We get fatter
- Allergies become more of an issue
- Plaque builds up on our arteries
- We sweat less
- We reduce muscle mass
- The brain shrinks
- Our teeth become less sensitive
- Our skin becomes thinner, less elastic and drier
- Our hair becomes less vibrant
- We get shorter
- The bladder becomes weaker
- Our heart activity slows down
- Our taste sensation is reduced
- Our hormonal activity changes
- Our bone density decreases
- We experience digestive system disorders

To offset these changes, we need to adjust how we eat. The key change is to reduce daily caloric intake, with a focus on vegetables, fruits, lean meats and fish.

2. Stress. Stress has a direct impact on our physical health, especially digestion and gut health. The best nutrients to reduce stress are:

- Potassium
- B Vitamins
- Calcium

- Omega-3 Fatty Acids
- Iodine

3. Dieting. Dieting is not the solution to long-term weight loss. When you go on a diet, the following things occur . . .

- Your metabolism slows down
- Your body kicks into fight or flight mode
- Your cortisol levels increase
- Stress levels rise
- You fixate on forbidden foods
- You tend to lose muscle tissue, water and minerals over fat

STEP TWO: CHANGING MINDSET

A powerful impetus to breaking free from the eating rules that enslave us is the concept of mindfulness. Mindful eating involves:

- Controlling what comes into the house
- Not allowing yourself to get too hungry
- Buying smaller plates
- Savoring your food
- Engaging all your senses
- Chewing your food thoroughly

- Slowing down

The two key hormones that regulate hunger are . . .

- Leptin
- Ghrelin

In order to balance these key hormones, you need to:

- Get 7-8 hours of sleep each night
- Eat protein with every meal
- Do regular exercise. High-Intensity Interval Training (HIIT) Workouts are ideal
- Eat more high fiber foods

The three parts of the Habit Loop are ...

- The Trigger
- The Behaviour
- The Reward

Remember, switching from a bad habit to a good habit doesn't have to require changing all three of these steps. If you stick with the same trigger and reward but simply switch out the action in the middle, you will be able to transform a bad habit into a good habit.

STEP 3: PRACTICAL SOLUTIONS

In Chapters 8 and 9, you were presented with dozens of practical tips, food recommendations and recipes to kickstart your nutritional transformation and establish your new, healthy nutritional habits. Some of these included:

Balance

You need to balance all 3 macronutrients in your nutritional plan. Carbohydrates, which provide glucose, are the most efficient energy source. Carbs also provide fiber, which promotes satiety and boosts gut health. Good health requires a balance of fatty acids, including saturated fats. Fats, in the form of triglycerides, are the major form of fat storage in the body. Protein, in the form of amino acids, makes up the building material of the body.

The Harvard Healthy Eating plate represents a good eating plan to follow. The key recommendations are . . .

- Fruits and vegetables: ½ plate
- Whole grains: ¼ plate
- Protein: ¼ plate
- Healthy plant oils: in moderation

Hydration

Water is essential to the efficient functioning of the body. Aim to drink 8 glasses of water each day. Sleep is also crucial to overall health, being especially important for renewing energy levels and relieving stress.

Recommended Maximum Daily Intakes

- Men should have no more than 30 grams of saturated fat daily.
- Women should have no more than 20 grams of saturated fat daily.
- No more than 5 percent of daily calories should come from sugar.
- Adults should have no more than 30 grams of sugar daily (7 sugar cubes).
- Adults should eat no more than 6 grams of salt daily.

Other Top Tips

- Add color to your plate by choosing vegetables that cover the rainbow. Eat at least 5 portions of a variety of fruit and vegetables every day. 2 fruit and 3 vegetable ideally.
- Do not classify food as good and bad. Instead,

separate them as either frequent or occasional selections.

- Eat some dairy or dairy alternatives (such as oat drinks); choosing lower fat and lower sugar options.
- Eat beans, pulses, fish, eggs, meat and other proteins (including 2 portions of fish every week, one of which should be oily).
- Avoid processed spreads like margarine and eat natural butter in small amounts.
- Foods high in fat, salt and sugar should be consumed in small amounts infrequently.

By putting all of this into practice, you'll no longer have to feel like a driver at the wheel of a runaway car. Those bad eating habits that you've been enslaved to for as long as you can remember will be things of the past, and you will be free to move forward with your new, better eating habits. Then you'll be able to wake up every day feeling that you are living inside of a well-maintained, tight machine that not only looks good but is functioning at its best. At the same time, you will have developed a new appreciation for food, relishing its nourishing properties and delighting in the abundance of exquisite flavor and variety.

You now have the power, so go and put it to use!

"Success isn't always about greatness. It's about consistency. Consistent hard work gains success. Greatness will come"

— DWAYNE JOHNSON

Thank you for purchasing 'Breaking Bad Eating Habits' If you have enjoyed this book, please leave a review on Amazon.

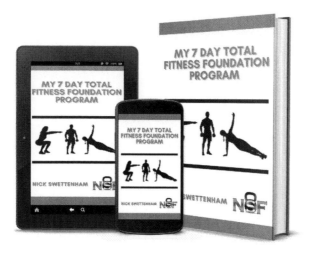

A Special Gift for my Readers

Included with the purchase of this book is My 7 Day Total Fitness Foundation Program to help you get started on your fitness journey. This program is a great way to start or adapt your training using all my 7 foundations. These foundations are:

1. Strength
2. Flexibility
3. Mobility
4. Stability
5. Agility
6. Endurance
7. Nutrition

Scan the QR code below and let us know the email address you would like it delivered to.

www.nickswettenhamfitness.com

REFERENCES

CHAPTER 1

https://www.sciencedaily.com/releases/2008/06/080630200951.htm#:~:text=FULL%20STORY-,Mothers%20who%20eat%20an%20unhealthy%20diet%20during%20pregnancy%20may%20be,to%20new%20research(1)

CHAPTER 2

Age-related decline in RMR in physically active men: relation to exercise volume and energy intake - v) PubMed (nih.go

https://pubmed.ncbi.nlm.nih.gov/18175749/

https://academic.oup.com/advances/article/3/
1/54/4644546

https://agsjournals.onlinelibrary.wiley.com/doi/full/
10.1111/j.1532-5415.2008.01732.x

Serum Lutein is related to Relational Memory Performance - PubMed (nih.gov)

Health benefits of anthocyanins and molecular mechanisms: Update from recent decade - PubMed (nih.gov)

Effect of a 12-Week Almond-Enriched Diet on Biomarkers of Cognitive Performance, Mood, and Cardiometabolic Health in Older Overweight Adults - PubMed (nih.gov)

CHAPTER 3

https://psychologyofeating.com/the-stress-metabolism-connection/

https://barbend.com/stress-strength-training/

https://www.healthline.com/health/stress/effects-on-body#4

https://www.healthline.com/health/cortisol-urine

Cholesterol in Eggs May Not Hurt Heart Health: Study
– WebMD

https://www.hindawi.com/journals/jobe/
2011/651936/

https://www.ucsf.edu/news/2004/11/5230/ucsf-led-study-suggests-link-between-psychological-stress-and-cell-aging

https://www.mayoclinic.org/healthy-lifestyle/stress-management/in-depth/art-20046037

https://www.ncbi.nlm.nih.gov/pmc/
articles/PMC3181836/

https://www.livestrong.com/article/460992-does-stress-increase-metabolism/

https://www.jneurosci.org/content/33/17/7234

CHAPTER 4

R. Cleland et al., "Commercial Weight Loss Products and Programs: What Consumers Stand to Gain and Lose. A Public Conference on the Information Consumers Need to Evaluate Weight Loss Products and Programs," Critical Reviews in Food Science and Nutrition 41, no. 1 (January 2001): 45–70, doi:10.1080/20014091091733.

CHAPTER 5

Effects of chewing on appetite, food intake and gut hormones: A systematic review and meta-analysis - PubMed (nih.gov)

Chewing and Attention: A Positive Effect on Sustained Attention (nih.gov)

https://pubmed.ncbi.nlm.nih.gov/24854804/

https://pubmed.ncbi.nlm.nih.gov/24854804/

CHAPTER 8

https://www.health.harvard.edu/staying-healthy/healthy-eating-plate

https://www.cnbc.com/2021/03/01/harvard-study-mix-of-fruits-and-veggies-linked-to-longevity.html

CHAPTER 9

https://fitfoodiefinds.com/healthy-pancakes-1-base-batter-6-ways/

https://www.delish.com/cooking/recipe-ideas/recipes/a51807/low-carb-breakfast-burritos-recipe/

https://www.wellplated.com/kale-feta-egg-toast/
#_a5y_p=3422321

https://simply-delicious-food.com/easy-healthy-salad-sandwich/

https://www.bbcgoodfood.com/recipes/spiced-lentil-butternut-squash-soup

https://www.bonappetit.com/recipe/bright-and-spicy-shrimp-noodle-salad

https://www.bonappetit.com/recipe/lemony-salmon-and-spiced-chickpeas

https://www.lecremedelacrumb.com/one-pan-spanish-chicken-rice/

https://www.acouplecooks.com/shrimp-and-broccoli/

https://www.jamieoliver.com/recipes/chicken-recipes/grilled-chicken-with-charred-pineapple-salad/

https://www.delish.com/cooking/recipe-ideas/recipes/a36265/steak-dijon-recipe-ghk0214/

https://glutenfreeonashoestring.com/homemade-protein-bars/

https://www.modernhoney.com/6-healthy-superfood-smoothies/

https://drivemehungry.com/sweet-and-tangy-sticky-soy-glaze/

OTHER BOOKS BY NICK SWETTENHAM

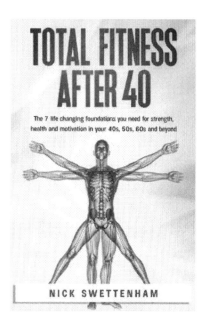

To purchase scan the QR code below

Printed in Great Britain
by Amazon